BORN TOO SOON

A Series of Books in Psychology

Editors
Richard C. Atkinson
Gardner Lindzey
Richard F. Thompson

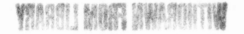

BORN TOO SOON
PRETERM BIRTH
AND EARLY DEVELOPMENT

SUSAN GOLDBERG

The Hospital for Sick Children, Toronto

BARBARA A. DiVITTO

Developmental Disabilities Unit
Massachusetts Mental Health Center, Boston

W. H. FREEMAN AND COMPANY
New York   San Francisco

Project Editor: Pearl C. Vapnek
Designer: Sharon Helen Smith
Production Coordinator: William Murdock
Illustration Coordinator: Richard Quiñones
Compositor: Graphic Typesetting Service
Printer and Binder: The Maple-Vail Book Manufacturing Group

Chapter-opening photographs:
Introduction, Chapters 1, 2,
3, 5, 6, Summary—Copyright ©
Suzanne Arms/Jeroboam, Inc.
Chapter 4—Copyright ©
Lawrence Cameron/Jeroboam, Inc.

Library of Congress Cataloging in Publication Data

Goldberg, Susan.
    Born too soon.

    (A Series of books in psychology)
    Bibliography: p.
    Includes index.
    1. Infants (Premature)   2. Child development.
3. Infants (Premature)—Care and hygiene.   I. DiVitto,
Barbara A.   II. Title.   III. Series.
RJ250.G64   1983   155.4$'$22   82-18381
ISBN 0-7167-1445-0
ISBN 0-7167-1446-9 (pbk.)

2 3 4 5 6 7 8 9 0   MP   1 0 8 9 8 7 6 5 4

Contents

Preface

From 1974 to 1978 we collaborated on a study that took us into the homes of preterm infants several times in the first year of life. From 1979 to 1981, one of us (S. G.) was engaged in a second study, in which preterm infants were visited at home twice a week for six months. In the course of these two studies, we got to know parents quite well and found that parents depended on us as part of their support system. Insofar as possible, we tried to meet parents' needs for information about their babies and early development. The one request that always made us feel helpless was "What can I read about the development of preterm babies?" Aside from the many technical, inappropriate journal reports, we knew of nothing we could offer.

It was in this context that the idea for this book was born. We realized that many families with preterm babies had generously contributed time and energy to helping us find out about the development of these infants in the home—that the information gathered could help other families in the future. We felt some obligation to repay this investment by sharing with parents what we, and others, have learned.

This is not a book about how to care for a preterm baby. Nor is it a book of advice or opinion. We believe that is best left to professionals who work with individual babies and families and have information about individual needs and strengths. This is a book about the unique experiences and problems of preterm infants as well as some of the ways in which they are similar to their full-term counterparts. We try to point out areas where there is wide variation among both full-term and preterm infants and some of the ways in which preterm infants may be especially difficult to care for even when their development is quite normal. We also identify the most frequent developmental abnormalities among preterm babies and how often these occur.

There is no crystal ball that can predict any baby's future. The infant development specialist, like the life insurance companies, can only "go with the averages." Here we try to make clear what the averages are for preterm infants and how they have been obtained. We have not tried to describe or summarize every study that has been done, but rather to select examples that illustrate particular themes, methods, or problems. Many important studies have therefore not been cited.

Although this book was written for parents, we hope that it will be useful to professionals who work with preterm infants and their families. Nurses who work in intensive care units for newborns and want to know what happens to the babies when they go home, pediatricians or general practitioners who don't see many preterm infants but want to give parents easily understood information and realistic expectations, and infant stimulation specialists who are seeing an increasing number of preterm infants are some of the people who may find this book useful. But most of all, it is for the parents who showed us it was needed and who have a right to know.

December 1982   Susan Goldberg
                                          Barbara A. DiVitto

Acknowledgments

Although we claim authorship of this book, many others participated in its development and completion. The research project that introduced us to the topic was funded by OCD grant No. 90-C-388, Biomedical Research Funds administered by Brandeis University, and a Radcliffe Fellowship to Susan Goldberg. The staff of that project, Sheila Brachfeld, Elizabeth Judd, Janet Leshne, Martha McKay, and Nancy Sheiman, made it possible for us to meet and understand the parents whose requests led to the decision to write such a book. However, it was only with the encouragement and assistance of Eric Wanner that we actually produced a manuscript.

Many colleagues read various versions of the manuscript and provided helpful reviews and suggestions, among them C. Zachariah Boukydis, Jeanne Brown, Tiffany Field, Edward Goldson, Arthur H. Parmelee, Nancy Shosenberg, and Marian Sigman. Lauri Lowen and Marian Ferguson provided reviews from the unique perspective of being both parents of prematures and professionals.

Verna Regan and the office staff in the Psychology Department at Brandeis University and later Eva

McGrath and the staff of the Word Processing Centre at The Hospital for Sick Children always produced the typed manuscripts on time. W. Hayward Rogers and the staff at W. H. Freeman and Company made the final stages of the process easy and pleasurable. We deeply appreciate the time and effort all of these people gave to turn a vague idea into the volume you now hold.

December 1982   Susan Goldberg
                                                 Barbara A. DiVitto

BORN TOO SOON

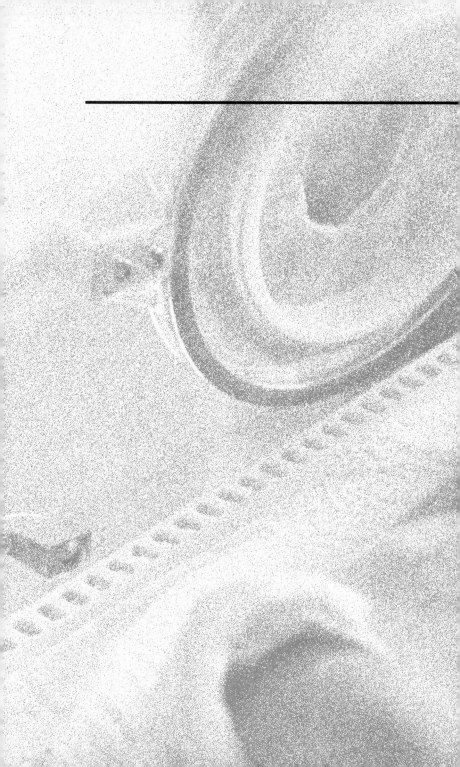

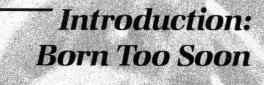

Introduction:
Born Too Soon

Judy is a bright, alert 4-year-old who has been in nursery school for a year now. She speaks clearly, moves with grace, and gets along well with her classmates. Both her parents and her teachers agree that she is normal, well-adjusted, and somewhat brighter than the average 4-year-old.

David is also 4 years old. He is an attractive, dark-skinned boy whose energy seems unlimited. In fact, his parents are somewhat concerned that he may be hyperactive because he has such a short attention span and seems unable to settle down at quiet periods like mealtime and storytime. Although he is difficult to manage, they have no other worries about his development.

In contrast, Martha is a 4-year-old who is a source of worry for her parents and her pediatrician. She has a serious motor handicap that prevents her from walking. Her speech is also affected. Though she seems alert, her speech and motor problems make it difficult to evaluate her real intellectual capacities.

3

Which of these three children was born prematurely? If you guessed all three, you are correct. Premature birth is the most common of all birth abnormalities. In the United States, 5–7% of all births each year (i.e., more than 150,000 babies) are premature. Most of these babies develop quite normally, others are mildly handicapped, and a few have lasting and serious problems. Of course, the same could also be said of children born after full-term pregnancies. What, then, is so special and interesting about premature birth that we should devote a whole book to it?

Obviously, something is considered special (and in this case worrisome) if it happens to you or to someone in your family. Premature births happen often enough that large numbers of new parents each year are affected. These parents wonder what they can expect in the future for their child. What are the chances that the child born prematurely will grow up to be normal? Although premature birth is associated with an increased risk for some handicaps, the actual incidence of such problems has been declining with improvements in early medical care and will probably continue to do so.

Indeed, the good news is that survival rates for preterm infants (those born before 37 weeks of gestation) are increasing, while the prevalence of problems is declining. Typically, the hospitals recognized as leaders in the care of prematurely born infants report in the early 1980s that 80–85% of the infants born before term at weights of 1000–1500 grams (2¼–3¼ lb) are surviving. Even more remarkable, 50–60% of the babies who weigh 750–1000 grams at birth (1½–2¼ lb) survive. Within these groups of the most fragile babies, about 11% are left with serious problems, such as blindness,

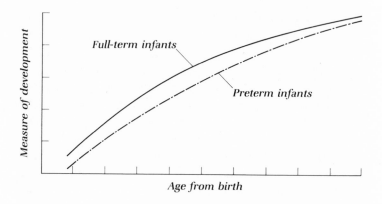

Figure 1 *Hypothetical growth curves for preterm and full-term infants.*

mental retardation, or cerebral palsy. Another 15% are moderately impaired by less severe forms of such handicaps, while the remaining 74% are normal or only very mildly handicapped.[1]

Thus, the majority of even the very smallest preterm babies will grow up to be normal in most respects. Though they differ in many respects from full-term babies in their early development, most of these differences disappear with increasing maturity. Figure 1 illustrates the typical pattern of development of preterm babies in comparison with full-term babies. The figure shows curves that could apply to several measures of development (e.g., weight, vocabulary size, improvement in motor skill) plotted against age from birth. What is clear is that both preterm and full-term groups reach the same level eventually. However, the preterm group gets there somewhat later.

For parents, of course, the nagging question "How will our child fare?" is a pressing one. Each family wants to know whether its baby will be one of the normal majority or a member of the handicapped minority. Because each child's situation is unique, no book can offer a reliable individual prognosis. Even the health-care professional who gives primary care to an infant and his family and knows the individual details has no crystal ball. What the health-care practitioner does is to make an educated guess, combining knowledge of the individual case with information about developmental outcomes among others with similar histories.

What this book can do is to provide some of the information that a skilled pediatrician, psychologist, or physical therapist would use in making an educated guess. Even more important, we try to provide realistic expectations of what parents will encounter in the first few years of development of an infant born prematurely—how preterm infants are like and unlike their full-term peers and how the experiences of parents of preterm infants differ from those of parents of full-term infants. Because parents play a vital role in providing the supportive environment and sensitive care for their baby that facilitates development, a summary of what to expect and look for can help them to understand and care for their preterm infants. In fact, there is considerable evidence that good care from parents in a stimulating environment is a powerful influence on the development of preterm infants and can overcome the potentially detrimental effects of early medical problems. This book is not meant to replace the judgment or advice of skilled clinicians, but to supplement it for those parents who want more information in a broad context.

Concern and interest in premature birth are not limited exclusively to parents. They are also related to controversies about the role of early experience in development. Does it have more powerful effects than later experience or not? Infants who are born early experience alterations in the earliest kinds of experience that we can study directly. Does premature birth significantly alter the course of their development?

One reason that the timing of birth is expected to influence subsequent development is that, normally, there is an optimal time for birth. If the infant were to stay in the uterus longer than the 38–42 weeks of normal, full-term gestation, there would be less room for further growth and movement, the infant might grow too large to pass through the birth canal, and the mother's body would be severely taxed to continue to meet the increased needs of the fetus. Indeed, there is some evidence that, after 42 weeks, the placenta (the organ that provides food and oxygen to the growing fetus and removes wastes) becomes less efficient in its work, so that babies born unusually late can be at a developmental disadvantage.[2] On the other hand, the fetus needs the support and protection of the uterus and placenta during the early and vulnerable period when the basic organs are being formed and until they are ready to function in the outside world. When birth comes too soon, the infant may not be capable of breathing, taking in food, controlling body temperature, and carrying out other bodily functions effectively and would ordinarily not survive.

A Brief History of Preterm Care[3]

The branch of medicine that includes disorders of the newborn, including prematurity, is called *neonatalogy* (which literally means "study of the newborn"). The first text in what we now call neonatology was written by Pierre Budin.[4] In it, he described the use of incubators, which he had designed for preterm infants in Paris. The modern descendants of Budin's incubators are in use in hospitals today and provide an environment in which temperature, humidity, and oxygen are carefully controlled. Budin's techniques for the care of preterm infants were brought to the United States by one of his students, Martin Cooney.

Cooney's career is probably most startling to modern medical practitioners because, during a large part of it, he was commercially successful at exhibiting preterm infants in their incubators at fairs and expositions in Europe and the United States. As late as 1932, Cooney's exhibit at the Chicago World's Fair was second only to Sally Rand, the fan dancer, in paid admissions.[5] It may be shocking to think that either parents or doctors would support his *kinderbrutenstalt* ("child hatchery") at the 1896 Berlin Exposition. However, the German doctors who provided the babies expected that the infants had no chance of surviving anyway. In fact, Cooney's demonstration of the success of new techniques in saving the lives of preterm infants was largely responsible for the adoption of these methods by American hospitals.

The first hospital center for the care of preterm infants opened at the Sarah Morris Hospital in Chicago in 1923. Many of the infants cared for had been born at home, as was common at the time, and then transported to the hospital for special care. A description of this nursery notes that "two or more wet nurses are required to supply the breast milk used in the station as all the young infants are fed, at least in part, with human milk."[6] Wet nurses received room, board, and $35 per month for their services.

However, a later report of this nursery cites overfeeding as a major cause of death among these infants, so that deliberate, early starvation became the rule.[7] For babies under 1200 grams (about 2½ lb.), the regimen was no feeding for the first 24–48 hours and then:

13th hour—1 tsp plain boiled water

15th hour—1½ tsp plain boiled water

17th hour—1 tsp breast milk

19th hour—2 tsp water

21st hour—1½ tsp breast milk

23rd hour—2½ tsp water

The babies were fed according to a 3-hour schedule by the second or third day.

We now know that this schedule does not meet the nutritional needs of newborns. But, in the 1930s, they were fed with bottles and medicine droppers and because swallowing and sucking were poorly developed skills or absent, a feeding could easily "go down the wrong pipe" and cause aspiration. For later and larger feedings, the technique of passing a tube to the stomach was just being developed.

Despite the limitations in techniques of care for preterm infants, of those who survived, 90% were in school in grades appropriate for their age.[8] However, at that time, only about half of all preterm infants were surviving. Today such a low survival rate applies to only the very smallest preterm babies, those under 1000 grams (2¼ lb).

Between the time that the Sarah Morris nursery started and the early 1960s, there were few major changes in the care of prematurely born infants. In the 1960s, however, neonatology really came into its own and became a recognized medical specialty. A technology that included more refined and varied techniques for assisting breathing, better equipment and laboratory tests for detecting physiological problems of newborns, new surgical techniques, new feeding methods, and new drugs began to make successful treatment of the special problems of preterm babies possible. Since the knowledge, equipment, and techniques for treating illnesses and problems of the preterm infant were highly specialized, very expensive, and useful for only a minority of births, it became difficult for every hospital to have its own unit for the care of ill or preterm newborns. Regional centers were therefore established to which babies from several local hospitals could be referred. This meant that methods of safely transporting these infants had to be devised. Today, a baby born prematurely on Cape Cod may be driven in a specially equipped van with a trained staff to a hospital in Boston for treatment. An infant born in Wyoming may be flown to a medical center in Denver for intensive care.

Since the 1960s, further refinements in medical

technology have dramatically increased the survival rate and decreased the number of problems found in preterm infants. The nature and organization of the care of preterm infants have changed in recent years and, to a large extent, medical technology has made it possible to solve the immediate problem of survival faced by preterm infants. Thus, the concern has shifted from sheer survival to the effects of preterm birth on subsequent development. Are some organ systems altered because an important part of their development occurred in an incubator instead of in the womb? Could it be that some systems (like hearing and vision), which are functional before birth, actually benefit from early exposure to the outside world?

While the new medical technology makes it both possible and necessary to ask such important developmental questions, it raises some of its own. Hospital staffs are very much aware that the time, money, and energy devoted to life support for preterm babies must eventually be evaluated not just in terms of how many lives are saved, but in terms of what the quality of life will be for these babies. Are the "miracle babies" growing up to be multiply handicapped youngsters and adults? To answer this question, many regional centers regularly follow these infants after they leave the nursery. The information that these follow-up programs have been collecting on large numbers of preterm babies over a long time period is what makes this book possible. Because most follow-up programs concentrate heavily on the first few years of life, this book does the same.

Who Is Born Prematurely?

As we try to trace the consequences of premature birth, it is helpful to know something about the cause of prematurity. Although we usually think about premature birth as the source of the problem, it is also a symptom or an outcome of previous events. It is possible that both premature birth and the infant's later development are traceable to a prior underlying problem. Much of what we know about the probable causes of prematurity comes from studies that ask who is born before term.

At least some instances of premature birth result from malformations and disorders associated with miscarriages, or spontaneous abortions. It has been estimated that only 31% of all pregnancies result in a live birth. There appears to be a natural selection process that results in miscarriage of the malformed or non-viable fetus. As medical technology saves younger babies, some may be the hardiest survivors of damaging conditions that would have resulted in miscarriage. These infants, of course, have lasting problems associated with the malformation that "caused" the premature birth. Fortunately, the number of premature infants who fall in this category is still quite small.

One kind of premature birth is caused by maternal health problems. Abnormalities in the mother's reproductive system may make it difficult or impossible for her to carry a pregnancy to term. Such malformations are relatively rare. Because pregnancy is so common and usually normal, we often forget that it makes great physical demands on the expectant mother. Any condition that adds to these demands or interferes with normal functioning increases the likelihood of premature birth. It is not surprising, therefore, that multiple births are often premature. A reproductive system designed to support one baby can support two or more for only a limited time period.

Chronic illness of the mother such as diabetes, high blood pressure, kidney or heart disease, can contribute to a shortened pregnancy. Ideally, such mothers with known complications of pregnancy receive careful medical supervision, so that the well-being of mother and child can be monitored. Often the decision is made to deliver such a baby early, before the health of the mother or baby is threatened. When such a decision is made, a planned early delivery will take place in a hospital that has facilities for the intensive care of newborns. In addition to those with known health problems prior to pregnancy, some mothers who were previously healthy develop problems because of the added stress of pregnancy. One reason for close medical supervision in normal pregnancies is to detect early signs of developing problems. In these cases also, a premature delivery may be deliberately planned.

General living conditions that adversely affect the mother's health, such as poor nutrition or inadequate medical care, make her more vulnerable to premature deliveries. Preterm babies occur more frequently among women of lower socioeconomic class, who live in less than optimal conditions and have less access to medical care. Mothers in disadvantaged groups of all kinds more frequently develop illnesses that complicate pregnancy.[9]

Pregnancies that occur before the reproductive system is mature or without adequate time for recovery between births are also associated with preterm birth. Teenagers under 15 are considered to be at high risk for preterm delivery. In part, this may reflect inadequate medical supervision of this group. Those who begin having children early and have many pregnancies close together are also more likely to deliver prematurely.

It is easy to see from these considerations why a mother who has had one premature birth is at higher risk than the average woman to have another one. Many factors that contribute to preterm birth do not terminate with the termination of pregnancy. They result from chronic health problems or from life patterns associated with chronic ill health. Furthermore, it is clear that infants born to such mothers are being reared in poor environments. These infants may be at a disadvantage socioeconomically and may have poor access to medical care.

In addition to physical problems, there is some suggestion that psychological stress may play a role in premature birth. The link is more tenuous, but it is one that obstetricians and psychiatrists have speculated about for quite a while. Much of the work on the effects of stress can be traced to the ideas of Hans Selye, whose work demonstrated that stress or tension in one body system can affect other systems.[10] Thus, prolonged psychological anxiety or tension may alter body chemistry and physiological functioning. Although this is an intriguing notion, we do not yet have evidence to document a strong relationship between stress and premature birth. However, the data we have on mothers living in disadvantaged conditions can also be viewed as indicative of the effects of stress.[11]

Despite this list of factors known or suspected to cause preterm births, about 50% of preterm births are unexpected and unexplained. That is, half of the premature infants are born after otherwise normal pregnancies of a physically healthy and emotionally stable mother who has had good medical care and is in her optimal childbearing years. It is common in these cases for parents to wonder whether they are responsible for the premature labor. They worry that maybe they shouldn't have taken a long car trip or had intercourse or allowed the mother to carry groceries in the days before labor began. So far as we know, there is usually nothing these parents could have done differently that would have prevented the premature birth. These parents need much reassurance from the medical staff that they have not caused the premature delivery. These infants are born without apparent malformations to mothers in reasonably good health who have adequate resources, good living conditions, and access to good medical care. These babies have the best opportunity for developing well—even if they were born too soon.

What Is the Prognosis?

What can we say about how most premature infants or the average premature infant turns out later on? First, we must note that, even at birth, there is an enormous amount of variation in the characteristics and experiences of those born prematurely. There is the infant who is born after a 37-week pregnancy and weighs 2500 grams (5½ lb) who is quite healthy—just small and immature. At the other extreme is the baby who is born after a pregnancy of 25–26 weeks and weighs 700–900 grams (1½–2 lb) who is very small, very immature, and vulnerable to such complications as respiratory difficulty and feeding problems, infections, and so on. While the first baby might stay in the hospital no longer than the average full-term infant, the second is going to have a prolonged, difficult course with a great deal of medical assistance and care. And, of course, there are all sorts of variations in the babies in between. Clearly, the prognosis for these two extreme cases will be quite different, but the same might be said for all the variations between them.

We do know that the younger and smaller a baby is at birth, the more likely the baby will have problems. This is partly because physical problems are greatest in the smallest babies and partly because such infants are often born to the most disadvantaged families.

As we noted earlier, changes in medical technology continue to bring about changes in prognosis. Thus, while some of the earlier studies reported that as many as 40% of preterm infants were afflicted with moderate to severe handicaps,[12] the current figure is more like 5–15%.[13] It appears that more and more of those born prematurely are blending into the general population. It is nearly impossible to walk into a preschool or an elementary school and identify those children who were born prematurely. The statistics on long-term outcomes for preterm infants born in the 1980s and later will be even more encouraging than those presented in this book.

Nevertheless, particularly in the early months and years of life, preterm infants are often markedly different from their full-term counterparts. In this book, therefore, we focus on the aspects of early development that may be distinctly different in the preterm group. However, "different" from the full-term baby does not necessarily mean "abnormal," especially for a preterm baby. In fact, we want to emphasize that what is "normal" for a preterm infant may be very different from full-term peers without heralding lasting deficits. For example, slow development is characteristic of preterm infants who have had major medical complications. They are, after all, recovering from serious illness and are hampered in behavioral development until physical recovery is complete.

As another example, we talk about ways in which preterm infants may be temperamentally difficult or frustrating for parents. "Difficult" here means more irritable or less responsive than the average full-term baby. While this makes life difficult for parents, it need not signify lasting social or emotional problems.

Thus, while we will often refer to ways in which preterm infants are less competent or more problematic than full-term peers in the early years, such statements must be viewed in the context of eventual outcomes that are predominantly normal.

Overview of This Book

The chapters that follow summarize what is known about the development of preterm infants. In Chapter 1, we begin by describing the early environment of preterm infants, the neonatal intensive-care unit (NICU). It is an environment that can be overwhelming and frightening to those who are not familiar with it, and it can be quite stressful to those who are. We try to explain the purpose of intensive care and some of the equipment and procedures that are a part of it. Chapters 2–4 describe the development of premature infants in various domains: cognitive, motor, and social. Chapter 5 examines the parents' experience of caring for a preterm baby. In Chapter 6, some of the many intervention programs that have been designed to help preterm infants and their families are described. In our concluding chapter, we provide a summary and evaluation of what we have learned about development through study of the prematurely born infant.

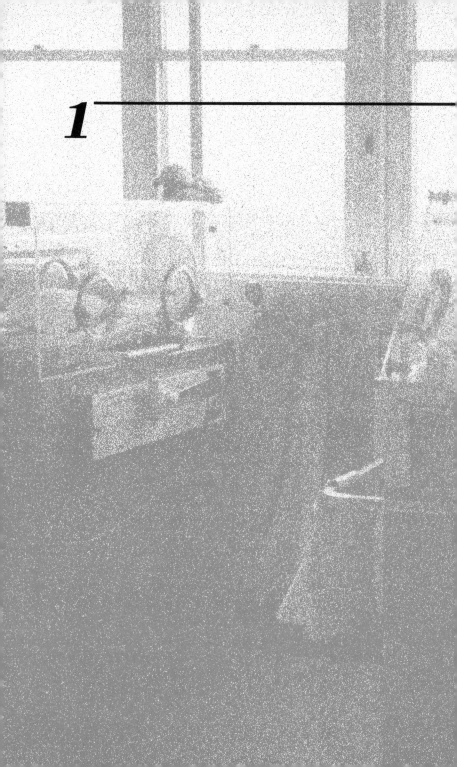

1

Early Days:
Intensive Care

The first sight of an infant in an intensive-care unit is usually quite distressing. For parents, whose expectations of "baby" were generated by magazine pictures of round-faced, rosy-cheeked 2-month-olds, it is even more disturbing. First, the younger the baby, the smaller and scrawnier she looks. Body proportions are different from those of a full-term infant. Perhaps even more disturbing than the actual appearance of the baby is how difficult it can be to see her at all. The incubator is usually surrounded by several pieces of strange machinery. Tubes and wires seem to emanate from every inch of skin. The baby's face may be partially covered by a blindfold to shield his eyes or a stocking cap to keep him warm. The nursery itself is filled with other babies looking equally "unbabylike" and with staff members engaged in frenetic activity. In this chapter, we try to describe this environment in which the preterm infant lives for days, weeks, or sometimes months, to explain the functions of this environment, and to consider its possible impact on psychological and behavioral development.

During the time an infant is developing in the uterus, many physiological functions are regulated or carried out by the mother's body. Although the infant's heart has been beating since about 2 months from conception, the circulatory system functions differently before and after birth. During prenatal life, the circulatory system includes vessels that go to the placenta, where oxygen and nutrients from the mother's body are absorbed and wastes are eliminated. The lungs do not function in respiration until after birth, and digestion is assisted by the mother's body. In addition, the mother's body maintains a constant temperature for the infant; systems for temperature regulation are inactive until after birth. The infant floats in amniotic fluid and does not have to work against gravity to move or support posture. There is little to see, but the sounds of the mother's voice, breathing, heart rate, and digestion provide much auditory stimulation for the fetus.

Birth brings about some very dramatic physiologic changes in the infant. Suddenly, the baby passes from this extremely supportive environment into one where all of his physiological systems must function effectively and independently. This is a stressful transition even for a full-term infant, and many of the behaviors that worry new parents reflect the inefficiencies of any newborn's physiology. Newborns sometimes breathe irregularly, hiccup, spit up, and often fall asleep during feedings.

When a baby is born prematurely, some physiological systems are not ready to operate. The lungs may not exchange gases or oxygenate the blood effectively. The infant may not be able to take food by mouth or to keep his body temperature up. Most of the problems encountered in the early days of a preterm infant's life originate in these physiological inadequacies. If the infant's organ systems cannot function properly, then surgical, mechanical, or chemical intervention must accomplish these tasks for him. In addition, the infant who cannot manage these bodily functions independently is also highly vulnerable to other problems, such as infections, breakage of delicate blood vessels (particularly worrisome if it occurs in the brain, called intraventricular hemorrhage), and lung disease.

Description of Intensive Care

There are two kinds of equipment and procedures surrounding the infant in intensive care. The first keeps track of bodily functions such as heart rate, breathing, blood-oxygen level, and temperature, so that the nursery staff will know whether and when the infant needs assistance. Many of these processes can be monitored continuously by a system that sounds an alarm if some limit is exceeded, for example, if the baby stops breathing (apnea) or if the heart rate slows suddenly (bradycardia). These systems are designed to ensure that someone will pay attention when something goes wrong. In addition, babies are weighed regularly, and urine, fecal, and blood samples are collected and analyzed on a regular schedule in order to manage fluids accurately. None of these kinds of equipment or procedures *influence* the baby's physiological functioning.

The second type of equipment or procedure assists or carries out bodily functions when the infant cannot do so alone. A plastic tube can pump extra oxygen into the incubator. A machine called a ventilator or respirator can assist the infant's breathing by pumping air through a tube that enters her nose or mouth and goes to the lungs. Food, medicine, and vitamins can be introduced directly into the bloodstream (intravenously) by insertion of a small needle into a vein in the hand, foot, scalp, or umbilical cord vessels. The infant can be fed through a tube that is passed through the nose down into the stomach (this is called gavage or tube feeding). A lamp producing artificial sunlight may be used to help break down bilirubin (a substance produced as old red blood cells are destroyed) when the baby's liver is not mature enough to do so. This condition, called jaundice (hyperbilirubinemia), may need to be treated by a blood-exchange process, which removes excess bilirubin from the baby's blood. Transfusions may be required for other problems.

All of this artificial management of the infant's bodily functions can create new problems. For example, in the early days of intensive newborn care, it was not known that exposure to high concentrations of oxygen intended to assist breathing could damage blood vessels supplying an important part of the eye (the retina).[1] Consequently, many preterm infants who needed respiratory assistance developed blindness (retrolental fibroplasia). Now that we understand that high oxygen levels are one cause of blindness, the administration of oxygen is monitored more carefully to avoid it. For example, a comparison of preterm infants cared for at the University of Colorado Medical Center in 1947–1950 with those treated in 1950–1955 under lower oxygen concentrations showed that, while the proportion of those with some retinal damage decreased only slightly (from 28% to 21%), the incidence of severe damage (blindness in both eyes) decreased dramati-

cally (from 13% to 1½).² Another example of a treat-
ment-caused (iatrogenic) problem is infection from
openings in the skin made to insert tubes or needles
for life-support purposes. Thus, the care of an infant
requiring a great deal of physiological assistance is quite
complicated.

It is not surprising that many parents report feeling helpless or useless in the face of the complex medical care their infant needs. However, it is important
to remember that all of the apparatus and procedures
are designed to meet the infant's physiological needs
during a time of crisis. Infants' psychological needs,
which parents are better prepared to meet, are tem-
porarily of low priority due to more pressing medical
needs. Nevertheless, this environment probably does
have psychological and behavioral consequences for
development. It differs radically not only from the womb
for which the preterm infant is ideally prepared, but
from the normal home environment for which she may
be partially ready. Before considering the possible psychological impact of these early experiences, we should
emphasize that each infant's actual experiences will
be different according to his age, weight, and special
complications.

Levels of Intensive Care

Thus far, we have talked about a variety of things
that may happen to a prematurely born infant. Some
infants have all of these problems, others have none of
them. The typical hospital unit for intensive newborn
care is organized into subunits that differ according
to the level of care required. One area is generally allot-

ted to those infants in incubators who need constant nursing or medical supervision. These include infants who need prolonged assistance with breathing, intravenous feeding, and continuous monitoring of many functions. In this area, a single nurse has only one or two infants in her care who are constantly watched.

At the other extreme are those infants who have recovered from early problems and are almost ready either to go home or to enter the regular hospital nursery. In this section, which some hospitals half-jokingly call the "grower room" or "pasture," there are also some infants who must be carefully observed because they are at risk for special problems since they are still small and immature, though they do not show any current signs of difficulty. Some healthy premature infants simply require extra investment in care and observation while they gain weight and strength. Here infants are in open cribs and are bottle-fed (or even breast-fed). There is little special equipment, and each nurse has several babies to care for.

Depending on the size of the unit, there may be one or more subunits for infants requiring different levels of intermediate care. As an infant's condition improves or worsens, he is likely to be moved from one subunit to another so as to best match his needs with the kind of care and equipment available.

The NICU as an Environment for Development

There has been a great deal of disagreement about the nature of the intensive-care unit as an environment

for preterm development. Those whose primary interest is in social or cognitive development think of the
complex social environment of a typical family and the
stimulation it supplies and describe the intensive-care
unit as a stimulus-deprived environment.[3] They point
out that there is little patterned stimulation, little relationship between the infant's behavior and environmental events, minimal social interaction, and nothing
appropriate to look at. Others, who are less concerned
with the kind of stimulation than its sheer amount,
point out that levels of sound and illumination are
high, that handling for routine care is frequent, and
that numerous people interact with each infant. Such
an environment may in fact be overstimulating rather
than understimulating the infant.[4]

Neither of these views takes into account what
the preterm infant is able or likely to respond to. Most
infants, even those born prematurely, have the ability
to shut out a great deal of unpleasant stimulation by
sleeping. Constant high levels of noise and illumination actually induce full-term infants to sleep, so that,
even though the environment itself provides high-
intensity stimulation, the infant may receive very little
of it. One pediatrician, who has done extensive research
with preterm infants, suggests that, until 35 weeks from
conception, the preterm infant's neurological system
is so immature that the environment has little impact
on it.[5] This view is still controversial. A more common
position rests on the fact that, during the last 6 months
of gestation and the first 6 months of postnatal life, the
brain and nervous system undergo a period of very
rapid growth.[6] Most texts in child development men-
tion this period as one during which the brain and

nervous system are especially vulnerable to outside influences. However, even if environmental conditions do not influence long-term development in preterm infants, we can ask what life is like for a baby in intensive care.

One careful study recorded sound and illumination levels in intensive-care units and grower rooms over several 24-hour periods.[7] Sound levels ranged from 60 decibels (the level of traffic at a street corner) in the grower rooms to 88 decibels (the sound in a motor bus) in the intensive-care rooms. (A typical business office produces sound levels of about 54 decibels.) All of these sounds were audible inside the incubators. In fact, the incubator and surrounding monitoring equipment produced much of the audible sound and accounted for the fact that the level and frequency of nonspeech sounds were higher in the intensive-care rooms than in the grower rooms. Speech sounds were also found with high frequency in the nursery during 83–88% of the observations. Though we have no comparable figures for a typical home, the fact that parents and siblings sleep for about 30% of the time indicates that infants in intensive-care nurseries are exposed to more speech than they would be in the home, even though most of it is not addressed to them. However, an understanding of the impact of such conditions depends on knowing how well preterm infants can hear—a topic that has not been well studied.

Fluorescent lights are on 24 hours daily in most intensive-care units. Where outside windows are present, solar light varies and produces some rhythmic day–night changes, less than in most homes. Since some nurseries are more heavily staffed during the day and routine care may be minimal at night, there may be rhythmic changes in levels of sound and frequency of handling, but these are likely to be less clearly defined than in home environments.

These considerations suggest that, in many respects, the preterm infant is exposed to more physical stimulation than her full-term counterpart at home. However, it is patterned differently, is less clearly rhythmic, and is unrelated to the infant's behavior or sleep–wake cycles. Rhythmic changes in patterns of stimulation may contribute to the developing infant's own rhythmic patterns of waking and sleeping, feeding and elimination. It seems that the reduced rhythmicity of the nursery does little to encourage the regularity in habits that parents long for in their young infant! This may be especially important for the baby who spends a long time in the intensive-care unit with a chronic problem.

There is a widely held belief that preterm infants, because they are fragile, should be handled as little as possible. However, routine nursing care, the collection of specimens for analysis, and care during medical crises often necessitate frequent handling. In the study described above, infants were handled during 11% of the observations in the grower rooms and 19% of the observations in the intensive-care rooms. In another study, which assessed the effects of handling on blood-oxygen levels, infants were handled at least hourly and sometimes more often for such matters as changing diapers or sheets, drawing blood samples, taking x-rays, and inserting or removing tubes.[8]

Regardless of the reason for handling, oxygen levels dropped with each intervention. Usually, infants recovered spontaneously, but sometimes respiratory assistance was necessary. Data such as these lead medical practitioners to believe that preterm infants should be handled as little as possible. All of these procedures are invasive and unpleasant. None was designed to comfort or soothe the baby.

A recent study has shown that 15 minutes of holding and cuddling three times daily, though it initially stressed preterm infants, resulted in increased oxygen levels over the course of a week as well as the ability to maintain oxygen levels during the holding periods.[9] This study suggests that handling designed to be comforting and pleasant for the baby may be less stressful than procedures considered medically necessary. The primary source of these more pleasant social experiences for infants in intensive care are parents and nurses (Figure 1).

In comparison to the infant cared for at home, the infant in intensive care is probably exposed to more frequent but also more unpleasant handling. In routine handling for medical and nursing care, there is generally little to encourage the preterm infant to look forward to social interactions. Nevertheless, nurses, when their routine duties allow them to, do engage in affectionate and playful interactions with the infants they care for. In fact, although there are no formal data on the subject, it is common for nurses in intensive-care nurseries to form attachments to the infants they care for. When asked to rate the attractiveness of pre-

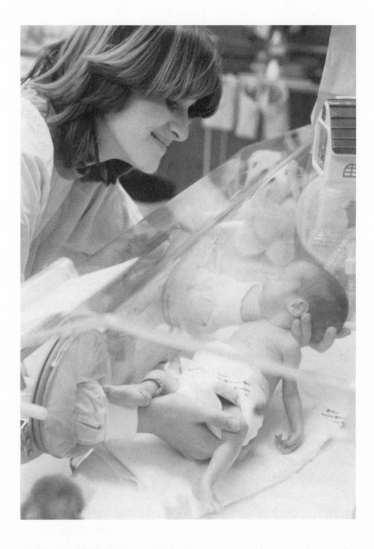

Figure 1   *During the hospital stay, some social interaction can be part of the preterm infant's experience. [Photograph copyright © Bob Stewart.]*

term infants from photographs, experienced nurses gave higher ratings to picture of babies they had cared for.[10]

Other nurses have described how depressed they feel when the babies to whom they have been giving primary care are well enough to go home. "I find myself crying on the way to work, knowing he has already gone home." A frequent pattern of behavior for many nurses is to wait a week or so before picking up another primary care baby after the previous one has gone home. Others want to begin caring for a new baby immediately. Parents may feel concerned about such attachments. On the one hand, they would like to be sure that someone is giving loving care to their baby when they cannot be there. On the other hand, they may wonder if they will be able to do as good a job as the nurse or fear that the baby will prefer the nurse to them.

One of the important differences between the interactions of nurses with infants and those of parents is that parents visit and interact only with their own baby while nurses may care for many babies. Conversely, each baby has only one set of parents, but may have many different nurses. One study found that, during an average stay in intensive care (49 days), a typical baby was cared for by 71 different nurses![11] Not surprisingly, nurse contacts tended to be briefer than those of the mothers. In another hospital, although nurses were the main source of contact for babies in intensive care, few of their interactions (other than feedings) lasted more than 9 minutes. Although cuddling was an infrequent form of interaction, it was one of the behaviors mothers were most likely to use and nurses least likely to use.[12] Thus, even during the period of intensive care, when parents are likely to feel that they cannot do very much for their baby, there is a special quality to parent–infant interaction that is not duplicated by nurses. Parents are likely to be more consistent figures in the infant's environment, and their interactions are longer and probably more comforting to their infant.

In recognition of this unique contribution that parents make, hospitals increasingly encourage parents to visit and care for their infants in intensive care whenever possible. Some index of the changing attitudes toward parents in intensive-care units can be obtained by contrasting the amount of parent visiting in a Cleveland hospital in the early 1970s with that reported from a Boston hospital more recently. In the first study, mothers who visited at least twice in three weeks were considered frequent visitors,[13] while in the second study, every baby had been visited daily.[14] Another recent study considered as frequent visitors parents who came four or more times weekly.[15]

Some infants are visited very little or not at all while in intensive care. Many of the reasons for infrequent visiting reflect the difficulties of traveling to and from the hospital. Most hospitals do not have intensive-care units, so that many preterm infants are transported from the hospital of their birth to a regional center with suitable facilities. This means that the mother is left behind and cannot visit until she herself is discharged. It also means that the father may have to choose between visiting the mother at a nearby hospital or the baby at a distant one. In some cases, even after the mother's discharge, visits to the intensive-care unit may not be feasible. The intensive-care unit at Children's Hospital in Denver, for example, serves an area that includes 10 states. Thus, the social experiences of infants in intensive care may vary a great deal even where hospitals permit and encourage visiting.

Apart from the effect of such visits on the baby, they are important to parents. It is especially difficult to feel like a competent parent when your baby is being cared for by medical personnel in an intensive-care unit. The accurate perception that the infant is having a stressful, unpleasant introduction to life can be very painful to parents. As one mother said, "... when I feel we are in tune, I feel like there is such rage there. After all, look what's being done to her—she is poked, prodded, hurt all the time. I feel the same way."[16]

If you have ever visited a hospitalized friend or relative under intensive care, you have some idea of the experiences of parents whose babies are in intensive care. However, remember that when you visit a relative or friend, it is someone you already know. When parents visit their preterm infant, they are trying to get acquainted with someone very important whom they don't yet know! Given the highly specialized medical equipment and procedures that abound, it is not surprising that parents feel anxious about how they will ever manage on their own, as well as upset or angry that their baby must be subjected to these frightening and stressful experiences. Thus, for the parents, the opportunity to contribute to the infant's care and comfort, to become familiar with the baby, to feel that they are special and important to the baby (rather than a less skilled substitute for a nurse or doctor), and to share these feelings with other visiting parents and with hospital staff are important steps toward taking responsibility for the exclusive care of their baby.

Although little is known about how the experience of intensive care affects later development, there is some evidence that specific procedures are stressful to the infant at the time they are carried out. Earlier, for example, we mentioned a drop in blood-oxygen level following routine handling. It may indeed be true that the neurological system is insensitive to environmental events until some late point in gestation—that these incidents have only transient effects.[17] However, most preterm infants remain at least in the grower rooms until they are close to term, that is, for several weeks after the 35- to 36-week gestational age at which some believe the infant becomes vulnerable. Of course, those infants with complications are likely to stay longer, and it becomes difficult to tell whether later developmental difficulties reflect the impact of the intensive-care environment or the problem that kept the infant there.

Policies for discharge vary widely among hospitals. In some, a healthy preterm infant whose parents are psychologically ready to take over may be sent home as soon as possible. In others, a specific age or weight must be reached before discharge is considered.

It seems safe to assume that all infants who spend time in intensive-care units are exposed to a unique and stressful environment. Many of the conditions are highly invasive, but considered necessary for the infant's survival. Those who care for infants in intensive care are increasingly aware of this; some of the efforts to provide a more supportive environment for infants and their parents are discussed in Chapter 6.

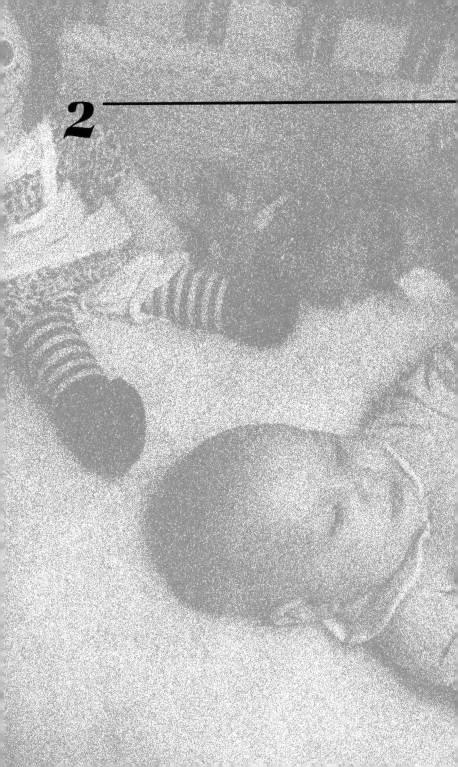

2

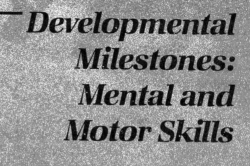

Developmental Milestones: Mental and Motor Skills

When something unusual, like early birth, has happened to their child, the first thing parents want to know after "Will he survive?" is "Will he be normal?" Whenever the question is asked, it usually reflects two primary concerns:

"Will our child have a normal IQ score?" (Will her mental skills be like those of age mates?)

"Is our child going to have serious difficulties in basic motor skills?" (Will she have cerebral palsy?)

These are indeed two of the areas in which those born prematurely are vulnerable to later developmental problems. For this reason, preterm infants, especially those who have had complicated medical problems, are usually evaluated regularly by means of developmental tests. In this chapter, we explain what such tests measure, what their limitations are, and what we have learned from such tests about the development of prematurely born babies. (Those who are not interested in the construction of tests can skip the next few sections and go to the bottom of page 51.)

Before a test can be devised to measure development, one must know what development is. The behavior of a newborn infant often seems to be a series of unplanned, uncoordinated accidents. There seems to be no organization at all. Certainly, it is less controlled than the behavior of adults and older children. Yet somehow, in a very short time, babies become those older children. The process by which these changes occur is what is meant by development, and a systematic catalog of the sequence and timing of those changes common to all human babies and children is one way of describing development. Most parents are familiar with many of these predictable changes as they eagerly wait for their baby's first smiles, words, and steps. Other changes may be less obvious to parents (for example, the changing pattern of grasping small objects as the infant makes the transition from using the whole hand and arm as a unit to the more precise one of the thumb and forefinger.) These landmarks or milestones of change are the basis of the most commonly used developmental tests. After many years of systematic baby-watching, developmental researchers have a great deal of information about the average age at which babies reach these milestones and how much variation is found among normally developing babies. For example, the average age at which babies begin to babble (repeat syllables such as *ba-ba, ma-ma*) is 5 months. But among normally developing full-term infants, it is not unusual for babbling to occur as early as 3 months or as late as 7 months. The average age for walking is 12 months, but may vary from 9 to 17 months in normal babies. Developmental tests take this information about developmental milestones and organize it in a way that allows us to assess the *rate* at which a baby is achieving these milestones. Thus, developmental tests are measures of the rate at which development is progressing.

Variations in Developmental Rates

There are wide variations in rate of development among normal babies. Some babies seem to be generally "fast" developers, while others come along at a more leisurely pace. Although all babies stand alone before walking, one baby may be taking a few steps at 11 months, while another makes few efforts until 18 months. All babies babble before they begin to say words, but some do both early and others do both later than average. Thus, when the average age for developing a particular behavior or skill is given, it may be masking vast differences in normal development. It is also the case that babies may be fast developers in some areas, slow in others, and about average in still others. Some babies seem to put more of their energies into one thing than another, and at different times different kinds of skills attract the efforts of the same baby. So one baby's motor abilities may increase rapidly, while his language skills might be coming along more slowly. Another baby seems most interested in other people and seems grown up socially, but may be slower than others in manipulating objects. These are all normal patterns of development, and it it is these kinds of differences that begin to contribute to each child's unique personality.

Some differences are probably inborn. Either through genetic inheritance or through some predisposing events in the uterine environment, babies may be born predisposed to fast, slow, or average rates of development. Some differences in rates of development probably arise from differences in temperament or interest. A baby who is active and eager to explore or one who is extremely persistent will probably acquire new skills more rapidly than a baby who is placid and slow-moving or one who is easily frustrated. A baby who is unusually fearful or shy may not take advantage of opportunities to explore or learn new skills.

Finally, development is influenced by the opportunities that are available for using new skills. Jean Piaget found that one of his children was quite delayed in the hand-watching that babies generally do in the 2- to 4-month period. Piaget recognized that much of this was attributable to the fact that this infant was born in the winter. He spent so much time bundled up in a snowsuit that his hands were not available for play. It is in this domain that the infant's environment can influence development. The baby who lies in a crib all day in a room without pictures, objects, or people has little opportunity to practice new skills. On the other hand, the infant who is constantly surrounded by toys and people and bombarded with continuous sounds from conversation, the radio, or the street may have so much to cope with that retreat to sleep is the only comfort. Opportunities are opportunities only when there is a good match between what an infant is able and ready to do and what is available.

Developmental Tests

While developmental tests identify those differences in rate of development that are within the normal range, their main function is to identify those babies whose development is progressing so slowly that it is not within the normal range. Most tests of infant development are similar in form and content and can be traced to the scales constructed by Arnold Gesell, a pediatrician who did very careful studies of infant development at the Yale Child Study Center in the 1920s and 1930s.

The basic idea of such scales is to collect a group of activities and tasks that represent the behavior of infants (0–3 or 0–2½ years) and can be ordered according to difficulty. Difficulty in this case is determined by the average age at which babies first succeed at a task. Something that generally occurs around 5 months of age (for example, looking for a fallen object) is considered more difficult than something that usually occurs at around 3 months (for example, hand play). Notice that, by this method, items can be ordered according to difficulty even when they assess very different skills.

When such an assortment of items has been generated and ordered, the next task is to present these items to a large sample of babies at different ages. Since the items are ordered by age, the older babies in this sample should succeed at more tasks than will the younger ones and, in general, as babies get older, they should systematically pass more items. The purpose of administering these items to a large sample (called the standardization sample) is to find the average number of items that babies at each age will pass. These averages then become the expected performance for babies at each age. For example, on the Bayley Scales of Infant Development, the average 4½-month-old is expected to pass 52 items, while the average 18-month-old is expected to pass 125.[1] A baby who passes more items than the average for his age is considered to be developing more rapidly than the average, while one who passes less than the average for his age is developing more slowly. The tabled averages also allow the examiner to estimate about how much faster or how much slower than average a baby is. Of course, few babies score exactly at the average for their age, and this is why the actual scoring takes account of the normal range of variation.

Since the standards or norms for development are based on the performance of the standardization population, it is important for that sample to be representative of the babies who are actually going to be evaluated. For this reason, norms established in one country may not be appropriate in another. In fact, there is some evidence that norms change over time.[2] When collecting data for the 1969 standardization of her scales, Bayley noted that the infants tested in 1958–1961 were more precocious than those tested for the previous standardization.[3] Others have also made similar observations in the 1950s and 1960s.[4] This change in normal performance may be attributable to inadequate sampling in the earlier standardizations or to changes in test procedures. It is also possible that cultural changes, such as improved nutrition and medical care or different child-rearing attitudes and practices, have influenced the rate of infant development.

One of the reasons that the Bayley scales are currently in wide use is that they are the most recently standardized tests, although they are based on data collected in the 1960s, which may now be "old." More recently, standardized tests have been constructed to evaluate the behavior of newborn infants, an age group that is not well represented on other scales. The most frequently used instruments for this purpose are the Brazelton Neonatal Behavioral Assessment Scales[5] and the Graham–Rosenblith scales.[6] Each of these includes simple tests of reflexes (such as sucking and the startle response) as well as responses to a variety of sights and sounds (for example, a ball, a rattle, the experimenter's face and voice) and routine caretaking maneuvers (being undressed, being picked up). Again, the scales are based on the typical performance of a large population of newborns on whom the test was standardized.

What Do Developmental Tests Predict?

The construction of infant tests is quite similar, in principle, to later tests of intellectual performance such as those typically used to obtain IQ scores. Nevertheless, it has been demonstrated over and over again that infant tests do not predict later IQ or school performance. In a general way, an infant who performs normally on infant tests usually performs normally at later ages. One who is extremely slow in early development often has a handicap that makes him a slow learner later on. In fact, infant tests are most successful at identifying those who will be seriously handicapped later on, but they usually cannot tell us, within the normal range, whether a child's tested IQ score will be 95 rather than 100, closer to 120 than 110. Why not?

First, the skills assessed on IQ tests (which are those required for success in school) are quite different from the behavioral repertoire of the infant. Why should smiling at a mirror at 5 months predict skill at reading and arithmetic? While we *can* predict that the infant who has not acquired the ability to discriminate shapes is not going to learn to read, we cannot predict from an infant's success at form discrimination how easily reading or arithmetic or other school skills will be acquired.

Second, for any group of normal babies who are similar in infancy, subsequent experiences will vary widely and there will be more variability in performance in the same group at, say, age 7. Another way to think about this is to imagine that infant tests predicted later IQ score or school performance perfectly. If this were so, regardless of what happened to them later on, a group of babies who obtained the same score at age 1 would also get identical scores or grades at age 7. Of course, we don't believe that. How well nourished a child is, how much attention and stimulation she gets from parents and siblings, and how much she has learned to value success in school are all viewed as important contributors to her later performance on IQ tests or in school subjects. Thus, the low predictive power of infant tests may be a reflection of the flexible nature of development and the ability of infants and children to respond to the experiences provided by parents and other caregivers.

We also need to keep in mind two other characteristics of infant tests. First, they measure only rate of development. Clearly, this is not the sole important aspect of development. Two 8-month-olds may be able to find an object hidden under a cup.

> *Janey intently watches the examiner hide a rubber bunny under a cup, immediately lifts the cup, retrieves the bunny with a gleeful smile, and begins to manipulate and examine it.*

> *Jeannie watches the bunny being hidden and has to struggle to lift the cup. When the bunny is revealed, she picks it up, glances at it briefly, and then drops it while she turns her attention to the examiner.*

Both babies would be credited with finding the bunny, but the qualitative differences in attention, persistence, and pleasure in problem solving are not captured by the test score. Yet these qualitative differences seem to reflect processes and skills that are important to our common-sense definition of intelligence. (In Chapter 3, we discuss other ways of studying mental or cognitive processes that capture some of these aspects of early development.)

Second, we have to remember that these tests rely very heavily on motor skills. Because babies can't talk or understand speech, it is hard to find out about possible internal thought processes. In using developmental milestones, we rely on what we can directly observe. But motor skills are, at first, also poorly organized. Most infant tests have a separate section for evaluating motor skills since these *are* important early abilities. But even items that are considered to present mental rather than motor tasks often require some motor ability (for example, finding a hidden object, putting pieces in a puzzle). Developmental tests do not distinguish between babies who fail to understand a task and those who understand but don't have the motor skills required.

Why Use Developmental Tests?

If these tests have so many limitations, why do we keep using them? First, because they are effective screening devices. When a child is consistently succeeding at age-appropriate skills, we can be reassured about his development. When a child's rate of development shows that he is delayed relative to age mates, this is a sign that further investigation is necessary to determine the reasons for the delay. Continued follow-up is then advisable to determine whether the delay is temporary or permanent. For the most part, a delay during the first few years of life, with which we are concerned here, occurs too early to be regarded as permanent.

Second, a skilled examiner has seen many babies in the same testing situation and can use this information to note whether there is anything unusual about an infant's behavior that might warrant further investigation.

Ruth, at 6 months, was not interested in any of the toys the examiner offered unless they were banged noisily in front of her. In the report to Ruth's pedia-

trician, the examiner noted this with the comment that Ruth might not be seeing as well as other 6-month-olds and that more specific visual tests would be useful.

Thus, the standardized developmental assessment, like the standard pediatric examination, provides an opportunity for a skilled clinician to compare the behavior of one baby with that of many others and to note atypical behaviors that may be indicative of problems.

Finally, these tests do give us a good picture of what a baby can and can't do at a particular time. It is on the basis of such evaluations of current functioning that most practical decisions are made.

Does this baby need more cognitive stimulation?

Does she need help with particular motor skills?

Would nesting boxes be a good toy to get now?

The fact that developmental tests do not predict later behaviors does not impair their usefulness as indicators of current abilities that can be used to make practical decisions.

How Old Is a Premature Baby?

Before we turn to some studies that have evaluated the development of preterm infants with standardized tests, it is necessary to decide how we are going to describe the age of a prematurely born infant. Remember that, on these tests, comparisons are being made between a baby and a standard population of age mates. When we consider prematurely born infants, we have to remember that, although we usually count age from the time of birth, all babies are not the same age at birth. A baby born after 40 weeks in the womb is older than one born after 38 weeks in the womb. In the life of a young infant (for example, a 1-month-old), two weeks is a long time. Ordinarily, we don't differentiate among full-term infants born on the early side of 38–40 weeks and those on the late side.

> *Amy, a prematurely born infant, spent only 30 weeks in the uterus. She was born 10 weeks earlier than most full-term babies. One month after birth, Amy is still younger than full-term infants at birth. If we were to evaluate Amy's development, would it make any sense to use, as the standard, babies who were 40 weeks from conception plus 1 month from birth when they were tested? Development really begins at conception rather than at birth, and we would not expect Amy, born after 30 weeks, to look or behave like average 1-month-olds a month after her birth. To whom should we compare her? A 34-week-old fetus? Other preterm babies at 34 weeks from conception? Probably the latter would be most appropriate.*

There are some normative data for preterm infants, but they are usually confined to neurological rather than behavioral evaluation or are designed to determine gestational age. For the most part, standardized tests do not include norms for preterm infants (although we will shortly demonstrate how norms for full-term infants can easily be adapted for this purpose). As a preterm baby gets older, it is possible to make comparisons with full-term infants born later.

About 10 weeks after her birth, Amy could be compared with full-term newborns; and 14 weeks after birth, she could be compared with full-term 4-week-olds. We can think about Amy's age in two ways. The first is her age from birth, or postnatal age. This is what we usually mean when we talk about age. The second way is to think of her age from conception, that is, how old she would be if she had been born on her due date (at term). When we do this, we are comparing her with full-term babies conceived at the same time. Thus, in Amy's case, since she arrived 10 weeks early, 10 weeks after birth she is at term; 14 weeks after birth, she is 4 weeks past term. We refer to this way of thinking about age as postterm age.

Other labels that have been used for the same purpose include "developmental age," "conceptional age," or "corrected age."

Early Development

Gesell strongly believed that development was largely a function of biological maturation. He expected that infants would develop on the same biological timetable regardless of the time of birth. Accordingly, Gesell prescribed the use of postterm ages when testing preterm infants.

We now have ample data to suggest that, for the most part, Gesell was right about the rate of development. Figure 1 shows performance on the Bayley scales for infants grouped according to how early they were born. Notice first that all of the curves have the same shape. This shows that the number of items passed is increasing at the same rate in all groups; that is, the rate of development, as measured by this test, is not affected by time of birth.

The second notable feature is that if we take some arbitrary score, say 80, and mark it on each curve, the age at which this point is reached is older and older as we look at babies born younger and younger. That is, we have to move further to the right on the age scale to find the point where the curve passes 80 on the vertical scale. The full-term group achieves a raw score of 80 on the Bayley scales at about 8 months. For infants born 3–5 weeks early, this score is achieved at about 9 months; for those 6–8 weeks early, this point occurs at 10½ months, and for those born 9–15 weeks early, the comparable achievement occurs at about 11½ months after birth. So a good way to get a rule-of-thumb estimate as to when a preterm infant can be expected to achieve developmental milestones is to look at the expected ages given for full-term babies, then use the preterm baby's postterm age rather than postnatal age.[7]

Figure 2 shows the curves as they would look if we used postterm age for the preterm groups (as opposed to age from birth, as in Figure 1). Notice that there is one place where the curves do not overlap as well as we would expect. Up to about 4 months of age, the preterm infants are getting better scores than are the full-term infants; moreover, the younger they were

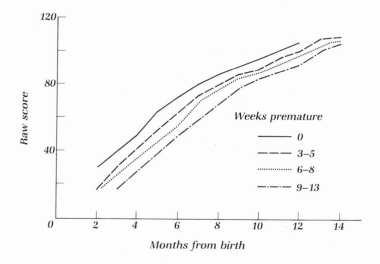

Figure 1 *Performance on the Bayley scales for infants grouped according to age from birth. [Hunt and Rhodes, 1977. © The Society for Research in Child Development, Inc.]*

at birth, the better their scores are. We found that this was also the case in our own study of preterm infants.[8] The fact that, in the first few months, early birth seems to give an advantage in test performance indicates that extra experience outside the womb may indeed enhance early development. However, this advantage is short-lived.

A similar pattern of development has been found for early motor skills: rate of development is not affected by the time of birth. However, the motor skills of pre-term infants are often delayed even when compared with postterm age mates. Typically, this extra delay is especially marked in the second half of the first year.[9]

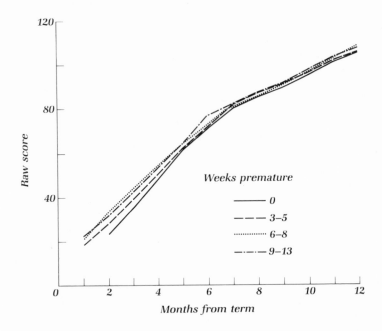

Figure 2 *Performance on the Bayley scales for infants grouped according to age from term. [Hunt and Rhodes, 1977. © The Society for Research in Child Development, Inc.]*

> *Amy, born at 30 weeks of gestation and tested at 8 months postterm, is likely to be performing like a full-term 8-month-old with respect to mental or cognitive skills, but may be more like a 7-month-old with respect to motor skills.*

One possible reason for delayed motor development is the period of forced inactivity during intensive care when the baby must lie in one position (usually on his back) for long periods of time.[10] Not only does this position prevent movements that would facilitate the development of muscle tone, but infants may come to prefer this position when it is no longer necessary and thus further limit their motor activities. They also may simply lack strength because recovery from their early illness is not complete.

This commonly observed lag in motor development, coupled with the heavy reliance of standardized tests on motor skills, suggests that these tests may consistently underestimate the mental abilities of preterm infants and that alternative methods should be used where possible. (In the next chapter, we discuss some of the methods other than standardized tests that have been used on a limited experimental basis.)

Later Development

One more feature should be noted in the two figures. All of the curves rise sharply at first and then slope more gradually. This is a pattern of all growth curves, whether they measure physical or behavioral functions: change is rapid at first and then slows down, eventually leveling off. If this is the case (and we can see that the curves don't continue long enough to tell), it is possible that the full-term and preterm curves may level off at the same place, even though the preterm curve reaches that level at a later point in time. Is this what happens? It is here that there is probably the most confusing array of findings.

Part of the reason for this confusion is that, as medical technology has changed, the outlook for children surviving preterm birth and its complications has

changed. Thus, earlier studies of children born prematurely paint a picture of long-term prognosis that
is too pessimistic for babies born in the 1970s and
1980s. In the earlier studies, as many as 40% of the
preterm births were associated with severe intellectual
and neurological problems,[11] while more contempo-
rary figures show a rate of 5–15% for these same problems.[12] In fact, technological change may be occurring
so rapidly that even a few years' difference in birth
dates may make a big difference in outcome. A recent
report compared preterm infants surviving respiratory
distress in the early 1970s with a similar population
born in the latter part of the decade.[13] The more recent
survivors obtained more optimal developmental scores
than had their counterparts born in the early 1970s.
Thus, while developmental impairment was once considered a common result of prematurity, it is no longer.

A second confusion is that there is great individual variation among preterm infants in age and weight
at birth as well as illness in the newborn period. Some
studies have included all babies born in a particular
hospital over a given time. Others have been restricted
to preterm infants with specific characteristics (for
example, those without complications or those who
received mechanical assistance with breathing). Still
others have compared different subgroups of preterm
infants. Each of these strategies provides information
about a different segment of the preterm population,
and differences in findings may reflect these population differences. Thus, one study may report no difference between full-term and preterm groups, and
another may report deficits among the preterm groups.
Careful inspection may reveal that the second study

had more preterm babies who had early illness or who were much younger and smaller than the first.

Most of the long-term studies of those born prematurely have used IQ tests as the main measure of how well the children fare later. These tests, as we pointed out, are constructed in much the same way that tests of infant development are. However, their main purpose has been to predict school performance, so the kinds of tasks and questions that appear on IQ tests are those that have been shown (in prior research) to be related to skills used in school. Like infant tests, IQ tests are standardized, so that children are scored in comparison with their age mates in the standardization sample. A score of 100 is assigned to children who are performing on the same level as their age mates. A score below 100 indicates that a child is performing less well than age mates, while a score above 100 indicates performance that is more advanced than that of age mates. How much above and below 100 is considered a real difference? A rough guideline can be taken from the norms established in the standardization process. About one-third of the children tested score between 85 and 100, while another third score between 100 and 115. This range, 85–115, which includes two-thirds of the population tested, is considered to be the range of normal performance.

IQ scores for children born prematurely generally fall within this normal range from the preschool years through middle childhood. However, when compared with groups of children born at term from similar backgrounds, the scores of the preterm group are typically slightly lower. For example, one study of 7- to 9-year-olds born prematurely obtained an average IQ score of 98.7, while the average score for the full-term group was 109.3.[14] In this study, as in others, individual variation in the preterm group was similar in amount and pattern to that of the full-term group. Findings such as these indicate that, when we look at measures based on rate of development (like IQ scores), the preterm group looks normal at preschool and school age. However, the pattern of this study is repeated in virtually every other follow-up report. Although both groups score within the normal range, the preterm group's average score is slightly lower than that of the full-term group. Thus, early birth does seem to be associated with some disadvantage in school skills, though the amount is quite small. Again, averages are only averages. Some preterm children in these studies obtain higher scores than those of full-term children, and some do worse.

Of course, rate of change is not the only important feature of development, even if it is the most frequently measured. When more detailed assessments of the quality of functioning are made, prematurely born children are found to have a greater incidence of difficulties than do their full-term age mates. For example, in the study reported above, at 7–9 years, children in the preterm group were more likely than those in the full-term group to have difficulty with tasks requiring visual and spatial skills (for example, copying a design using multicolored blocks). In a study of 5-year-olds, about half of the preterm group were found to have problems with auditory or visual skills (for example, discrimination, memory).[15] Among children 4 years of age, another study noted a greater incidence of behavior problems, as reported by parents.[16] Other problems with higher rates among the prematurely born include reading disabilities and poorer school performance than among age mates.[17]

Predictions About Later Development

One of the intriguing problems for developmental psychologists is whether, among children considered to be at risk for later developmental problems because of premature birth, we can predict which ones are most likely to have later problems. This question is, of course, of practical interest since early identification of developmental problems allows for early efforts at remediation.

As we mentioned in the Introduction, a small proportion of preterm births is associated with genetic defects and congenital malformations. These are usually identifiable, and some of the long-lasting effects of such anomalies are known. However, among those with no obvious pathology, can we predict developmental outcomes? Although we cannot make specific predictions about individual cases, the presence of certain characteristics or the occurrence of particular hazardous events is known to increase the risk of later developmental problems.

In general, those infants born younger and smaller experience the most frequent and severe complications and are most likely to suffer subsequent impairment. For example, in two relatively recent studies, follow-ups of infants who weighed less than 1500 grams at birth found that about 15% scored below 85 on IQ tests.[18] However, as is always the situation when we look at individual cases, some very small, young preterm children experience few or no complications and develop normally.

> *Robert is such a baby. Born after a pregnancy that lasted 26 weeks, he weighed 910 grams (2 lb). His 10-week hospital stay was uneventful and, except for one cold, he has not been ill in his first year. When we first saw him at 6 months postterm, he was a small, wiry, attractive baby and quite active. Although his fine-motor coordination was poor, he succeeded in doing most of the things that full-term 6-month-olds do on the Bayley scales. A month later, he was crawling and, by 10 months (post-term), he was walking with support. At 11½ months, he was walking alone, and he is the only baby (pre-term or full-term) in our recent study who was walking at 1 year. He began imitating words and actions around 10 months postterm. For example, he would wave and say "bye-bye" in imitation. By 11½ months, he was spontaneously using words like "bye-bye," "mama," and "no" appropriately. At his 1-year assessment, his performance on the Bayley scales was at the 15-month level, comparable to his postnatal age. At this time, we have no worries about his future development.[19]*

It is also easy to pick out, from our own experience, a baby who has not done as well as Robert even with more time in the womb and a more substantial birthweight.

*Jean was born after a 30-week pregnancy and
weighed 1370 grams. During her 9 weeks in the
hospital, she spent 4 days on a respirator when she
was having breathing problems, but had no other
complications. When we first saw her (at 6 months
postterm), she was a small, wide-eyed, but rather
placid baby. She was sitting with support, and her
fine-motor skills were limited. Her Bayley performance was comparable to a full-term 4½-month-
old. She began to crawl soon after 11 months (postterm), but had not yet begun to stand at the end
of the year. At that time, although she was babbling, she had not begun to imitate or use words.
Her Bayley performance was like that of a full-term
9½-month-old. Although Jean continues to develop
and acquire new skills, she seems to be falling further behind her age mates, rather than catching
up as Robert has done. She is a child for whom
we have concerns about future development. Thus,
in spite of her apparent advantage in age and weight
at birth, she has not done as well as Robert.*[20]

The point of these examples is that, even though
the youngest, smallest babies at birth are at greatest
risk for subsequent problems, there are exceptions.

Increasingly, the evidence has shown that single
measures, events, or complications are not good predictors of long-term development. Consequently, many
currently working on this problem feel that predictions are best made by getting as much information as
possible about each child through repeated assessments. This information is then combined into some

kind of cumulative index that is adjusted after each new assessment. Such an index includes information about the pregnancy and delivery, age and weight at birth, complications in the newborn period, medical and behavioral assessments, and the home environment.

One such system obtained 14 different measures for each infant in the first 9 months.[21] These included scores based on obstetric history, pediatric examinations at birth and at 4 and 9 months, visual-attention tasks at term and at 4 months, standardized tests of infant development (the Gesell scales), and home visits. On each of these measures, the baby received a score indicating how poor, average, or optimal his situation was. These scores were all based on 100 as the average, expected score. As each new assessment was completed, it was averaged with the others to indicate whether the infant's outlook was poor (less than 100), average (around 100), or optimal (above 100). Thus, a baby who was intially considered at risk because of many obstetric or postnatal complications may eventually be scored as average or even optimal if other conditions such as rapid recovery, a good home environment, or competence in early developmental tasks compensated for these early problems. Similarly, a baby who, though premature, had no early complications and a seemingly optimistic prognosis may later be rated as being at risk because of failure to gain weight, persistent illness, or poor care from parents.

The scores obtained after all the assessments had been done were then used to predict developmental status at age 2 and 5.[22] In addition, statistical analyses were done to determine whether some of the measures were better predictors (that is, more strongly related to the evaluations made at age 2 and 5) than others. One of the most interesting findings of this study was that assessments of the home environment and of the quality of the parent–infant relationship were better predictors than was information about birth, delivery, or other early medical events.

While this finding might, at first, seem surprising, it has been duplicated in other research.[23] It also makes good sense if we bear in mind that most early medical events are relatively brief, and it is quite possible that their effects are transient. On the other hand, the quality of the home environment and the parent–child relationship represent conditions that endure for a long time. Thus, a baby who is young and small and has had prolonged respiratory distress is certainly going to be better off going home to a secure, supportive home with competent parents than if she goes to a stressed family where the mother is ill or overworked or where other major problems such as unemployment can distract parents from infant care. In fact, in a supportive and stimulating environment, this baby will probably be better off than others who were older and healthier at birth, but go home to a poor or disorganized family environment.

A series of studies based on the home visits made in the study described above has reported that, within this large preterm sample, the infants who received more frequent care and more sensitive social responses from parents performed more competently on cognitive and language skills at 1, 2, and 5 years of age.[24] For example, infants whose mothers responded to their vocalizations by consistently vocalizing back showed more rapid acquisition of language skills. These find-ings are quite similar to those with full-term infants showing that good care and appropriate stimulation from caregivers provide the conditions for optimal development. Thus, in this respect, preterm babies, in spite of their early problems, can be helped by good care from loving, attentive parents.

3

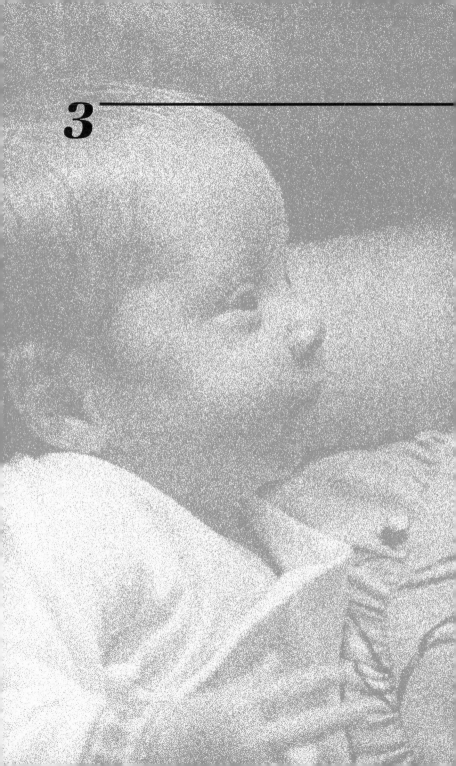

New Study Methods: Seeing, Hearing, and Exploring

Thus far, we have talked only about rate of development in achieving familiar milestones. While the milestones approach to development provides a description of behavioral change, it tells us little about the underlying processes that account for these changes. We could say that this approach is concerned with the *products* rather than the *processes* of development. The present chapter focuses on current methods of studying perceptual and cognitive processes in prematurely born infants. (We wish that such a chapter could also be written about motor processes, but the information in this domain is still too meager.)

As long as the predominant view of development focused on milestones, it was common to view infants as passive, helpless, and not very skilled. After all, the list of milestones they have not yet reached is very long. As soon as we began to look at perceptual and cognitive processes (for example, discrimination, memory, attention, and learning), we realized that infants are very competent indeed. Even in the first few days of life, the full-term infant demonstrates the capacity for selective attention, memory, perceptual discrimination, and learning. For example, in one study, breast-fed infants while still in the hospital showed that they could "recognize" the odor of their mother's nursing pad in contrast to one worn by the nursing mother of another baby.[1] When the two pads were hung one on each side of the infant, the babies turned toward their own mother's pad more often than toward that of the unfamiliar mother. In order to detect this ability, it was necessary to make detailed observations of infant behavior in a carefully structured and controlled laboratory setting. In the last 20 years, researchers have become increasingly sophisticated about designing such laboratory experiments, and the remarkable catalog of infant skills has been rapidly expanding.

One impetus to the acceleration of research with infants was the discovery that patterns of infant attention could tell us a great deal about infant perception and cognition.[2] The method used to make this discovery was to present the infant with two visual stimuli side by side and to record the direction and duration of the infant's looking. If the infant looked at one target more than at the other, he could be said to be capable of distinguishing them. This visual-preference technique showed that infants prefer patterned to plain surfaces, moderately complex to simple patterns, and novel patterns to familiar ones. Armed with this knowledge, we could ask all kinds of other questions:

> How long does an infant need to look at something before it becomes familiar?
>
> How much change in a pattern makes it novel?
>
> Are some properties of patterns more salient than others?

Two methods for varying novelty and familiarity have been commonly used. The first is a variation of the visual-preference technique. One stimulus is presented for a single long exposure (or familiarization period), and then it is paired with a succession of other stimuli that vary from it in systematic ways. Another technique provides many repeated brief exposures of the first stimulus. During these repeated presentations, infants typically show a decline in attention. Just like you and me, infants become bored and inattentive if the same thing happens over and over. If a new stimulus is then presented, infants typically perk up and pay attention again. To be sure that the change in response is specific to the new stimulus and not to irrelevant changes in physiological state (such as increasing hunger or fatigue), the familiar stimulus may be presented again. This procedure is often called the method of habituation (because it depends on the infant becoming accustomed to or habituating to repetition) or the discrepancy method (because it asks whether the infant notices discrepancies in procedure when a new stimulus appears). The technique assumes that attention declines with repeated presentation because the infant builds up the expectation that the same event will occur each time. Once the event has become familiar, the infant attends only long enough to make sure it is indeed "the same old thing." When change is introduced, the expectations of the baby are violated; attention increases again because the infant tries to find out what the new event is. Notice that this approach assumes that the infant actively tries to make sense of the surrounding world.

In both these methods, careful selection of stimulus materials enables us to find out what features infants notice and remember. By varying the duration of exposure, the time between exposures, and the delay between the presentation of the familiar event and that of the novel event, we can study the time course of infant memory processes. In addition, although static visual stimuli have been the most frequently used, a stimulus may be presented in other sensory modes (hearing, smell, touch) and can be complex and dynamic (for example, a voice repeating a sentence, a moving object passing behind a screen and reappearing). The infant's response need not be looking; it can be head-turning, sucking, heart rate, movement patterns, and the like. Thus, although these methods require complex experimental designs and laboratory equipment, they offer a wide array of alternatives that can be adapted for testing infants and children with motor handicaps or specific sensory deficits.

Development Before Term

Let us go back now to the time immediately after birth, when the preterm infant will have had 3–15 weeks of extrauterine life before reaching the developmental state of the full-term newborn. Studies of preterm infants during this time can tell us something about normal development before birth. Comparisons at term among infants who have had different amounts of postnatal experience can also tell us something about the effects of extrauterine, as opposed to intrauterine, experience.

One consistent finding in studies of these very young infants is that there seems to be an important change in behavioral and neurophysiological organization around 35–36 weeks from conception. First, patterns of waking and sleeping become more clearly defined at this time, although they still differ from those of full-term newborns.[3] Second, there are concurrent changes in visual attention. Although visual attention has been noted as early as 30–31 weeks of age and there is some evidence of the ability to make simple discriminations at this time,[4] the more common observation is that blank stares and poor coordination of the two eyes predominate.[5] However, from 35–36 weeks on, alert expressions and active scanning are observed,[6] and discriminations based on features such as brightness, black–white contrast, size, and number of pattern elements are similar to those of full-term newborns.[7] Although more controversial, there is evidence of change in the response to auditory stimuli at this time. Reflexes such as sucking and rooting have become strong and are more readily elicited.[8]

It is such evidence, coupled with experimental work on neurological development of the visual and auditory systems in animals that led to the notion that the effects of experiences prior to 35–36 weeks of age may have little effect on neurological development in human infants.[9]

Seeing, Hearing, and Touch

If early postnatal experience does influence maturation, then preterm infants who were born earlier should show more mature behavior at term than do those born later. (The previous chapter reported a small effect of this kind.) The baby born at 30 weeks' gestation will have had 10 weeks of postnatal experience when she reaches term, while the baby born at 35 weeks will have had only 5 weeks outside the womb at the same age. In contrast, the average full-term baby will have had, at most, a few days of postnatal experience when observed before discharge from the hospital. When we make such comparisons, we have to be careful to temper our naturally optimistic belief that "experience" is a good thing. Experiences in the intensive-care unit may be detrimental rather than beneficial. Or the infant may not be able to take advantage of the experiences. Younger babies may have more complications than do older ones, and the energy a preterm baby needs to maintain physiological functions (such as breathing, temperature control, and digestion) may be diverting energy normally available for maturational processes during growth in the uterus. Thus, it is not clear that more postnatal experience is advantageous to the infant born before term.

One study showed 28 preterm and 28 full-term infants a checkerboard target when all were 40 weeks postconception.[10] On the average, the first look of the preterm infants was twice as long as that of the full-term infants (12.89 versus 5.98 seconds). But is longer looking a more mature or less mature behavior pattern?

One way of thinking about this is to regard the ability to sustain attention as a developing competence. The infant whose looking pattern is immature and disorganized might just take occasional, short, unsystematic looks, while the infant with more mature skills might engage in a long period of systematic scanning. With this thought in mind, the above data seem to indicate that preterm infants do have an advantage over full-term infants in the ability to sustain attention. However, in general, researchers have found that, in the early months, older infants spend less time looking at a pattern than do younger infants.[11] In addition, with repeated presentations of the same pattern, older infants show a more rapid attention decrease than do younger ones. Thus, amount of looking seems to reflect how quickly or efficiently infants can take in the information in a visual target. A shorter look indicates more rapid information processing.

With this in mind, we can return to the study described above and surmise that the longer looking in the preterm group probably reflects a poorer or less-organized response to visual information rather than a more mature one. This interpretation is supported by other data from the same study showing that overall attention over three presentations of the checkerboard decreased more rapidly in the full-term group (from 21 to 11 seconds) than in the preterm group (from 30 to 21 seconds).[12] However, among the preterm infants, those who had more postnatal experience (that is, were born younger) tended to spend less time looking at the target. Thus, although overall the preterm infants seem to show less mature patterns of attention than do the full-term group, those preterm infants with more experience tend to show more mature looking patterns.

Other studies of visual behavior using the preference technique suggest that the ability to discriminate targets on the basis of form, size, and number of elements develops in preterm infants at the same time as in full-term infants of the same postterm rather than postnatal age, indicating that postnatal experience has no effect on these skills.[13] One exception in this group of studies was preference for three-dimensional rather than two-dimensional faces, a task in which experience seemed to accelerate preferences in the preterm group.

In these studies, "experience" is used in a vague and general sense to mean whatever happens to the baby after birth. We already know that preterm infants can have vastly different experiences. One way to explore the effect of specific experience is to provide a planned routine of stimulation. In one study, half of the preterm infants received a daily massage, soothing talk, and rocking for a period of about two weeks during their hospital stay.[14] At 6 months postterm, the group that received this treatment performed as full-term infants on a preference-for-novelty task; that is, they preferred the novel stimulus. The remaining preterm infants did not prefer the novel targets. However, in a second part of this study, a nonstimulated group of infants who were given twice as much time to become familiar with targets did show a preference for novelty, as did the stimulated preterm group and the full-term group. This study, like the looking study described earlier, suggests that preterm infants are less efficient than their full-term counterparts at processing visual information. It also indicates that a specific kind of soothing experience improved these skills. (In a later chapter, we give other examples of stimulation programs designed to enhance early development in preterm infants.)

Unlike vision, where we can depend on looking to tell us how much attention a baby gives to a target, hearing and touch are more difficult to test. Once again, we can use the idea that if a baby responds differently to different stimuli, he has discriminated among them. The behaviors most often used to evaluate hearing and touch are changes in body movement, breathing pattern, and heart rate. It is also possible to record electrophysiological changes in brain activity in response to auditory stimuli (auditory evoked potentials). This seems to be a promising method for early identification of hearing loss, which is estimated to affect about 1 in 50 infants who have been in intensive care.[15]

A recent study compared heart-rate responses of preterm and full-term infants to repeated presentations of pure tones.[16] The preterm infants in this study were 35 weeks postconception, while the full-term infants were 5 days postterm. Both groups of infants showed heart-rate decreases when the tones were sounded. However, the full-term infants showed less and less response with repetition and a bigger response to a new tone, but the preterm infants did not become accustomed to the tone (habituate) with repetition or respond differently to the new tone. Thus, 5 weeks prior to term, preterm infants do respond to sounds, but do not seem to process and use this auditory information in the same way that is typical of full-term newborns.

Most of the studies using auditory and tactile stimulation with preterm infants have studied responses during sleep. When sleeping full-term newborns are presented with a brief sound, such as a rattle, or a light stroke on the stomach, they briefly move their limbs in response and show a quickening heart rate. If the sound or touch is repeated several times, these responses usually disappear, demonstrating the infant's ability to shut out experiences that disturb sleep. When this same kind of stimulation is presented to preterm infants at term, they seem to need stronger stimulation to give a response (a louder sound or a heavier touch) but, once they have responded, they continue to respond on successive presentations without being able to shut out the interfering stimuli.[17] In addition, while limb movement and heart-rate response are closely related for full-term infants (that is, babies who show more movement also have greater heart-rate change), this is less true for preterm infants. Preterm infants were also characteristically found to have a higher resting heart rate than did full-term infants and to make less vigorous behavioral responses.

These differences suggest that, at term, preterm infants are less sensitive to sound and touch than are full-term infants. Their higher resting heart rates may indicate (as we suggested earlier) that they exert more energy in taking care of their internal needs and are less available to respond to external events. However, once they respond, preterm infants seem less able to shut out interfering stimuli and return to a sound sleep. Since these studies were done during sleep, they also suggest that the sleep states of preterm infants are somewhat different from those of their full-term counterparts, which is borne out by other studies of waking and sleeping behavior.[18]

What these studies illustrate is that preterm infants often show an uneven pattern of development. While they occasionally do seem more mature than their full-term counterparts in the early months (for example, their preference for three-dimensional faces), there are other respects in which they are less mature (for example, processing repeated visual information) and still others in which they are like full-term babies of the same postterm age (for example, form discrimination). In the latter instance, experience seems to have no effect. In other studies, experience before term seems to have a detrimental effect (for example, the preference for novelty), and, in still others, it has been shown that specially designed experiences can have a positive effect. The answer to the question of whether experience before term can affect development seems to be: It depends. It depends on what aspect of development one examines, and it depends on what one means by "experience."

In order to determine whether experiences before 35–36 weeks' gestation have less effect than those that occur later on, it would be desirable to assess the effect of a specific experience administered for equivalent amounts of time at different ages from conception. In most of the studies we have described, "experience" was used in its more general sense to mean "postnatal life." The actual experiences of infants born before 35–36 weeks' gestation were probably quite different from those of infants born at older ages. Thus, it seems that a definitive judgment on this issue cannot yet be made.

In thinking about these studies we should also remember that investigators are reporting group averages. Even when the preterm group has performed less well than the full-term group, there are usually babies in the preterm group whose performance is similar to that of full-term infants. Determining which babies account for the group's poorer performance and whether they share any important characteristics is important for the development of diagnostic tools. At the conclusion of this chapter, we return to this issue.

Exploring and Playing

As infants get older, we are less dependent on visual behavior and nonspecific measures like limb movement and heart rate for information about infant skills. Many of the techniques used to study visual attention in early infancy have been adapted to the study of manipulation and exploration of objects in older infants. Just as preterm infants show less preference for novelty on a looking task, they later explore novel objects with their hands less than do full-term infants at the same developmental stage.[19] Often, these findings are reported to be more characteristic of babies whose previous histories place them at higher risk for later developmental problems.

Infants' responses to novel objects are studied by allowing them to play with a toy for a set period of time (analogous to presentation of the visual target in the looking studies). Then the familiar toy is paired with a novel one. One interesting variation of this method set out to determine whether infants who had handled an object without seeing it would treat it as a familiar object when it was presented visually.[20] In order to do this, the infant has to translate information received in one sensory mode (tactual) into another sensory mode (visual). At 1 year of age, full-term infants were able to do this and attended more to the novel object (that is, the one they hadn't handled). At the same postterm age, preterm infants did not seem to recognize the familiar object. There are several possible explanations of this finding. One is that poorer motor skills in the preterm group limit the amount of tactual information they can obtain. Alternatively, preterm infants, as less efficient information processors, may need more time to become familiar with the handled object, just as they needed more time to look at the visual target. Finally, preterm infants may indeed lack skill in combining and comparing information from two sensory modes.

There are other examples suggesting that, in their play, preterm infants do handle and explore objects differently than do full-term infants at the same post-term age. As we watch babies explore objects, a developmental pattern can be observed.[21] When infants first succeed in reaching for things, the objects ususally go directly to the mouth. To the dismay of hygiene-minded parents, the first explorations take the form of sucking, biting, and chewing. Soon after the middle of the first year, banging, then shaking, throwing, and examining an object that is being manipulated appear in the infant's repertoire. Activities that combine objects, such as putting blocks in a container, appear toward the end of the first year. At first, objects are combined in ways that have little to do with their functional uses (for example, a spoon is likely to be banged against a cup rather than used to stir something in the cup or spoon things out of it). Functional use of toys appears early in the second year. Still later, toddlers begin to pretend with toys in ways that allow them to substitute objects for others in play.[22] For example, a toddler lacking a toy cup may pretend to drink from a shell. This systematic progression in play seems to reflect increasingly complex cognitive abilities, and observation of play may therefore be used to make inferences about developing cognitive skills.

One researcher watched preterm and full-term

infants freely handling objects.[23] At 8 months postterm, the preterm infants used the same kinds of
manipulations as did the full-term group, but there
were subtle differences. Preterm infants spent more of
their time looking at objects, while full-term infants
put objects in their mouths more often. In our own
study, we found that preterm infants who had had
early respiratory problems did less mouthing than did
postterm age mates. However, we also found that the
full-term infants frequently alternated mouthing and
examining objects, while the preterm infants rarely
combined activities in this fashion. In addition, we found
that, in a floor-play situation, at 8 months postnatal
age, the respiratory-distress preterm group spent less
time engaged with the toys than did the full-term group.
At 12 months, although the amount of time spent in
play was similar for these two groups, only the full-
term infants engaged in activities that combined objects
such as putting blocks into a container, putting rings
on a peg, or banging two toys together.[24]

Predictions About Later Development

These studies suggest that preterm infants, particularly those who have had other complications in
the newborn period, are less actively engaged in
exploring objects than are full-term infants of the same
postterm age. Much of the information summarized
here suggests that this *may* reflect subtle deficits in
information-processing skills or in sensory integration.
We also need to remember that these play activities

depend on manipulative skills, in which preterm infants are likely to lag behind their full-term peers. However, both researchers and clinicians are interested in finding out whether assessments of cognitive and perceptual processes are related to later difficulties of those born prematurely. The area that has received most attention in this respect is that of visual acitivity.

Partly because looking has been an easy behavior to record reliably, partly because looking is one of the few behaviors young infants can control, and partly because vision plays such an important role in human behavior, vision has been the most intensively studied sensory mode in both adults and infants. It also seems to be one area in which early abnormalities are predictive of later developmental problems.

Several studies have found that newborns who did not attend to moving objects were more likely to have visual–motor difficulties at 8 months and to have motor problems at age 4.[25] Babies who were unusually sensitive to light were also more likely than the average baby to have developmental deficits at 1 and 4 years of age. A more recent study found that, in a sample of at-risk newborns, many of those whose patterns of visual attention were characterized by blank stares, random scanning, or failure to attend to the target were identified as retarded or abnormal in their second and third years.[26]

Thus, the study of looking behavior seems to hold some promise for the early diagnosis of developmental problems. Some of the other techniques described in this chapter may also prove useful in this respect. Surely these approaches seem more closely related to the problems in speech, hearing, and attention expected to appear in a small proportion of the school-age children born prematurely than the standardized tests of infant development. While the latter rely on measuring rate of development, the newer techniques come closer to evaluating qualitative aspects of individual differences in specific skills.

Nevertheless, it is important to exercise caution in using early behavior that is typical or normal in preterm infants as a clear sign of an unfavorable prognosis. One physician–psychologist describes what he calls "iatrogenic retardation."[27] What happens in cases of iatrogenic retardation is something like this: The pediatrician anticipates a poor developmental outcome for a child and conveys this expectation to the parents. The parents lower their expectations for the child's development and because they expect little, they provide few challenging experiences. Consequently, the child does little. Thus, the anticipation of a poor outcome can become a self-fulfilling prophecy. In his own work, the physician–psychologist who recognized iatrogenic retardation has demonstrated to parents by alternative assessment techniques (like those described in this chapter) that their child does have age-appropriate cognitive skills. The effect of such a demonstration is usually to generate an enthusiasm in parents that is soon translated into rapid developmental gains for the child.

A recently published volume of studies based on the follow-up of preterm births reviewed four reports made when the children were 2–10 years old.[28] It noted that condition at birth (birthweight, age, or illness) had only small effects on later outcomes, while environmental factors (such as parents' educational level or social class) were the best predictors of later development. One of these studies included measures of visual attention and object play such as those discussed in this chapter.[29] These measures were found to predict development at 2 years of age mainly because they were related to measures of infant care: Infants who differed in visual attentiveness were treated differently by caregivers, and caregiver–infant relationships were better predictors of 2-year status than was visual attention. Thus, even when these more experimental assessments of cognitive skill predict later development, they do so less well than measures that reflect the quality of home care.

While early identification of developmental delays can be useful for early remediation, it can also ensure an unnecessarily poor outcome, and predictions from infancy can be unreliable. For this reason, it seems more useful to concentrate on the meaning of the findings in the present chapter for the current treatment and care of preterm infants. Knowledge of the ways in which "normal" preterm infants differ from full-term infants enables parents and other caregivers to form realistic expectations of current behavior and to use such expectations to guide immediate interactions with the infants in their care. It seems to us to make the most sense to respond to each child in terms of what she does (rather than what she cannot do) and what she is like now (rather than what she might become). It is also much safer since we often can't predict reliably what someone may become.

4

Individual Differences: Personality and Socialization

This chapter addresses the question:

> To what extent, if any, are temperament, person-
> ality, and social skills influenced by preterm birth
> and its accompanying stresses?

Although the idea that the first few years of life play a
formative role in personality has long been accepted,
the study of early individual differences has been much
less popular. After all, the argument went, babies and
toddlers don't do very much, so there isn't much scope
for individual differences. Parents, of course, have always
been quick to form firm impressions of each baby's
individuality: one baby is placid and easy-going, another
is difficult and irritable, a third is strong-willed and
stubborn. Whether these parental impressions are
accurate or not, the image a parent has of his baby
probably influences the care a baby receives. Thus, as
we consider the early social skills and temperament
of preterm infants, we can ask two questions:

> Do preterm infants as a group share any unusual
> characteristics?

How do these characteristics affect relationships with adult caregivers?

In this chapter, we concentrate primarily on the first question and address the second in the next chapter.

Although it may seem strange to think of a young baby as having social skills, those who have studied infant behavior and adult–infant interactions have been impressed and fascinated by the extent to which infant behavior, characteristics, and skills seem to be designed to ensure that adults will be especially interesting to babies, that babies will easily capture adult attention, and that adults and babies will get along easily. For instance, Konrad Lorenz, an ethologist noted for his studies of aggression in animals, was the first to point out that the appearance of young infants in many species is characterized by a cluster of features that adults find appealing.[1] These include a large head, flat nose, broad cheeks, large eyes, and smooth, soft body surfaces (Figure 1).

In addition, even the limited behaviors of young infants have a strong effect on adults. Smiles and cries are good examples. Any parent who has spent a sleepless night trying to quiet a crying baby knows how controlling the cries of a baby can be. For most adults, the impulse to pick up a crying baby is quite strong and, indeed, controlled research studies indicate that this is about the most effective way to quiet a crying infant.[2] Rocking or bouncing the infant, another frequent adult response to crying, is another.[3]

The smiles of a young baby can be equally powerful—and certainly more pleasant. Who among us has not at one time or another engaged in an otherwise

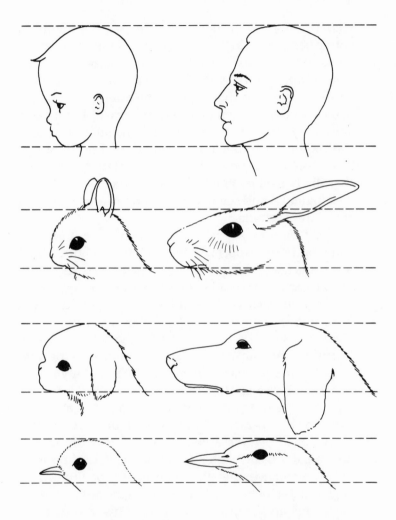

Figure 1 *Comparison of visual features provided by morphological characteristics of infantile and adult forms of four different species: human, rabbit, dog, and bird. While the infantile characteristics release parental responses, the adult ones do not. [Lorenz, 1943.]*

embarrassing performance for the sake of getting a young baby to smile? The exaggerated antics that adults perform for babies—head nodding, exaggerated facial expressions, and baby talk—capitalize on exactly those stimulus qualities that capture the attention of young babies: movement, change, and contrast.[4] It has been suggested that these particular behaviors and skills evolved because they enhanced survival of offspring.[5] While this view is not universally accepted, it does seem that the behaviors and skills of infants and adults are well matched and seem to be biased toward facilitating social interactions.

Let us now see how the preterm infant fares in some of these respects. When an infant is born before term, it is likely that some of the characteristics of full-term infants have not yet developed. In Chapter 1, we pointed out that preterm infants look quite different from full-term infants. Because they have not had a chance to add the layers of fat that give the full-term infant a soft, rounded appearance, most young preterm infants appear thin and scrawny. Many of the babyish characteristics that Lorenz pointed out are not prominent in preterm infants (Figure 2). Thus, they may look less attractive to adults than does the average term baby. However, appearance isn't everything. You may recall from Chapter 1 that nurses found preterm babies attractive after they had cared for them. This suggests that behavioral experience can certainly overcome this apparent disadvantage. (This is something most of us discover in our adult friendships as well: people "look" different to us after we have known them a while.)

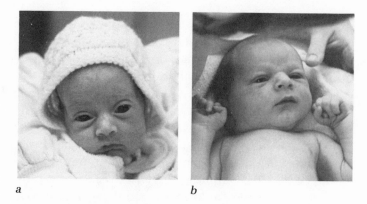

a   b

Figure 2 *The preterm infant's face (a) is less round than that of the full-term baby (b). [Photograph a copyright © Bob Stewart. Photograph b copyright © Suzanne Arms/Jeroboam, Inc.]*

Social Smiles

In the newborn or neonatal period, babies do smile, but these very early smiles seem to be unrelated to events that adults associate with smiling. The early smiles tend to be very brief, to take place when the baby is asleep, and to occur without social stimulation. Researchers sometimes call these reflex smiles, or endogenous smiles, since they appear to be caused by internal rather than external stimulation. Most adults dismiss such a smile with "It's only gas." Preterm infants often seem to exhibit more of these reflex smiles than does the typical full-term infant, although we don't really know why.

What most adults call "real" smiles are those that occur in social situations: when face to face with a partner, with eye contact, and in response to a partner's behavior or to an interesting physical event. In full-term infants, these smiles first appear at 6–8 weeks of age. The onset of social smiling is thought to be primarily determined by maturation because the time of occurrence is so universal. Blind babies, for example, begin smiling at the same age as sighted babies, even though visual stimulation is one of the main cues for smiling.[6] We would then expect that preterm babies would begin social smiling when they reach term plus 6–8 weeks. However, at least one study has found that babies born prematurely engage in social smiling earlier than expected—adjusting for about 50% of the degree of prematurity.[7] Thus, for a baby born 10 weeks early, social smiling would be expected to appear at 6–8 weeks after term minus 5 weeks (that is, 11–13 weeks after birth). However, in this study, special efforts were made to elicit smiles. In another study, when mothers were asked to report when their babies began social smiling spontaneously, the age of first social smiles for preterm infants was indeed term plus 6 weeks.[8] Thus, it seems that the spontaneous emergence of social smiles is not affected by experience under typical circumstances. This means that parents of a preterm baby have a long time to wait for the excitement and reward of social smiles.

Cries and Irritability

Unlike smiling, crying is a behavior that occurs from birth onward, and this is true for preterm babies as well. Because crying is such an important signal, it has been intensively studied. One of the interesting features of cries is that they carry information about the health of the infant. The cries of babies who have been physiologically stressed during prenatal development actually sound different from those of healthy newborns.[9] They are higher in pitch and have a different timing pattern. The cries occur less often and only in response to more stressful stimulation. This is the case for infants who are small for gestational age or whose mothers had complications of pregnancy and delivery, and it is also true of preterm infants.

The ordinary adult also recognizes that these cries sound different. In one study, parents of infants were shown videotapes of a preterm and a full-term baby in quiet and crying states.[10] A dubbed sound track was used so that each picture could be paired with the full-term and the preterm infant's cries on separate trials. In order to assess adult reactions, changes in heart rate, blood pressure, and other physiological changes were recorded, and a questionnaire was administered. The cries of the preterm infant elicited more of the physiological changes associated with stress than did those of the full-term infant. In addition, on the questionnaire items, the cries of the preterm infant were judged more unpleasant and irritating than those of the full-term infant.

Apart from the sound quality, how much a baby cries, under what conditions, and how easily a baby is consoled are important kinds of early individual differences. The Brazelton Neonatal Behavioral Assessment Scales include items that ask these questions about newborn crying. Several recent studies of preterm infants have evaluated their performance on these scales. A consistent finding is that preterm infants, especially those who have experienced respiratory distress, cry less during the examination than do their full-term counterparts.[11] Although some of the examination procedures are mildly stressful (for example, being undressed, being tested for reflexes), preterm infants cry less during these procedures than do the full-term comparison infants.

Many parents of preterm infants have confided to us that at first they worried because their infants didn't cry much. This concern is a sensible one: cries are the main attention-getting signal of young infants when they need help. Why do preterm infants cry so little during behavioral examinations? Two suggestions have been made. The first is that it takes a great deal of energy to cry, and preterm infants (as we have suggested before) may not have enough energy to cry. The second is that, for those infants who have been in intensive care, the behavioral examination is so much less stressful than many of their previous experiences that they are better able to tolerate its mild stresses than their more fortunate full-term counterparts. The first suggestion is given some support in the above studies by the finding that, along a continuum of general activity level (or arousal), preterm infants spend more time in the drowsy and sleep states, while full-term infants spend more of the examination time shifting among different waking states (quiet, alert, active, and crying).

Observations of preterm infants at later ages consistently show them to be fussier or to cry more than full-term infants in similar situations. In our own study, when we repeated the Brazelton newborn behavioral assessment 10 days after hospital discharge, we found that, from the first to the second assessment, the full-term infants had become less irritable, while the pre-term infants had become more irritable.[12] In addition, in four feedings we observed over the first four months, the same pattern was noted: the full-term infants grew less fussy as they got older, while the preterms became more fussy.

Studies of still older preterm infants also report that they are more irritable and fussy than the full-term comparison group. Field conducted a study in which mothers and their 3½-month-old infants were engaged in face-to-face social play.[13] Preterm infants were less attentive to their mothers and fussed more than the full-term infants. A second study, by Craw-ford, reported a similar pattern (greater fretfulness in preterm infants) during home observations at 6, 8, 10, and 14 months after birth,[14] and we found this to be the case during floor-play observations at home and in the laboratory at 8 months.[15] Parent ratings of 4- and 8-month-old infants on the Carey Temperament Survey (a questionnaire designed to evaluate infant temperament) also confirm this.[16] Mothers of preterm infants describe them as irritable and difficult to console more often than do mothers of full-term infants.

Are there any explanations for the seemingly greater irritability of older preterm infants? One possibility, which led us to predict in our study that preterm babies would be more difficult and irritable than full-term infants, is that this simply reflects the higher level of family stress associated with premature birth. A second possibility is that part of this greater fretfulness, especially among the older infants, reflects the immaturity of preterm infants. By the end of the first year, most infants have decreased their crying as they develop other means of communication. In fact, in Crawford's study, when preterm infants at 8 and 10 months postbirth were compared to full-term infants at 6 and 8 months, the differences in fretfulness disappeared, indicating that immaturity did contribute to the irritability of the preterm group.[17] However, in two of the other studies this was not the case: preterm infants were more irritable than full-term babies of the same postterm age.[18] However, in both of these studies, the preterm infants in question had all had respiratory complications, while in Crawford's study healthier newborn histories were more numerous.

For a small group of infants who have chronic lung disease after hospital discharge, extreme irritability can be a direct consequence of their medical problems. These babies (who have bronchopulmonary dysplasia or BPD) for several months after they go home, cannot get enough oxygen to feel comfortable, even when they are in no physical danger. They tire very easily and become irritable after only a short wakeful period. As their lungs become more healthy, they also become less fussy.

Yet another possible explanation occurred to us as we watched our 8-month-old group of preterm infants in the floor-play situation and evaluated their development. You may recall from Chapter 2 that preterm infants often experience a lag in motor development greater than expected from their immaturity alone, while this is less true of mental skills. This fact suggested to us that preterm infants may often wish to accomplish things, such as retrieving a toy or manipulating an interesting object, but lack the motor skills to do so. This would be extremely frustrating and could be yet another reason for the irritability that has been reported.

Alertness and Responsiveness

A number of other observations, some from the studies discussed above and some from studies discussed in previous chapters, should also be noted as temperamental characteristics of many preterm infants. In Chapter 3, we noted that preterm infants are less responsive than full-term infants to some forms of stimulation. This is corroborated by ratings on the Brazelton scales, on which preterm infants typically obtained poor scores on the social-interaction items, such as the ability to stay alert and to respond to face, voice, rattle, and ball.[19] This is also true when mothers were asked to rate their infants on the same items.[20] Mothers of preterm babies gave them poorer scores than did mothers of full-term infants.

In addition, it is typically reported that, regardless of the task assigned, preterm infants seem to be less actively involved than are their full-term counterparts. In a study of face-to-face play, preterm infants not only fussed more than the full-term group, but also were less attentive to their mothers.[21] A study of feeding behavior found that preterm infants were less active than full-term infants.[22] In our own feeding observations, we found that, of the time the nipple is available, full-term infants spent a larger percentage of it sucking

than did preterm infants[23] and, in our free-play observations, they spent more time playing with toys than
did the preterm group.[24] Another study also found
that preterm infants played with toys less often and
spent more time looking around than the full-term
group.[25] This was one group difference that was not
explained by immaturity. During standard developmental assessments on the Bayley scales, our staff rated
the preterm group as being less task-oriented, less persistent and spending more time looking and less time
manipulating objects than did the full-term infants.[26]

Attachment to the Caregiver

One of the major tasks in an infant's social development is the formation of a special emotional bond
with at least one caregiver. Typically, this happens
around 11 months of age. The experimental design
most often used to assess the infant's attachment, usually to parents, is called "the strange situation."[27] It is
a series of episodes involving the infant, a parent, and
a stranger, in which each adult enters and leaves the
room, leaving the infant alone or with the other adult.
Some of the most common reactions of a securely
attached infant include free play and exploration in
the presence of the parent, some inhibition of these
activites when the parent leaves, wariness when alone
with the stranger (contrasted with interest and even
approach when the stranger appears in the parent's
presence), and happy greeting when the parent returns.

In contrast, insecurely attached babies may explore very little in the parent's presence and show ambivalence or avoid the parent at reunions. They may also be more willing to accept the stranger as a substitute for the parent.

Several studies of premature infants have employed the strange situation to measure attachment.[28] None has reported any unusual characteristics of preterm infants. Just as with full-term babies, most of the preterm infants examined were securely attached to their mothers. As with full-term infants, about one-third of the preterm infants were insecurely attached.

Predictions About Later Development

There have been few reports of later personality and social skills of children born prematurely. One study reported that, at preschool age, there were few differences between full-term and preterm infants in social skills, as assessed on the Vineland Social Maturity Scales.[29] This is a brief inventory based on parents' reports of preschoolers' self-care in dressing and feeding and of responses to social situations. However, parents of preterms in this study did report more minor behavior problems such as poor attention span. Another study observed infants in a nursery-school setting at age 3.[30] There was some evidence that the children who had been born prematurely were rated as less socially competent with peers and teachers than was the full-term group. These findings do not yet form a cohesive picture, mainly because there have not yet been enough follow-up studies on social and personality development.

In summary, it seems that, in the early months, a number of characteristics combine to make the typical preterm baby somewhat more difficult to get along with. However, in many respects, such as the quality of attachment to the mother and some social skills, the evidence so far suggests that preterm infants do not differ after the first year from their full-term peers.

5

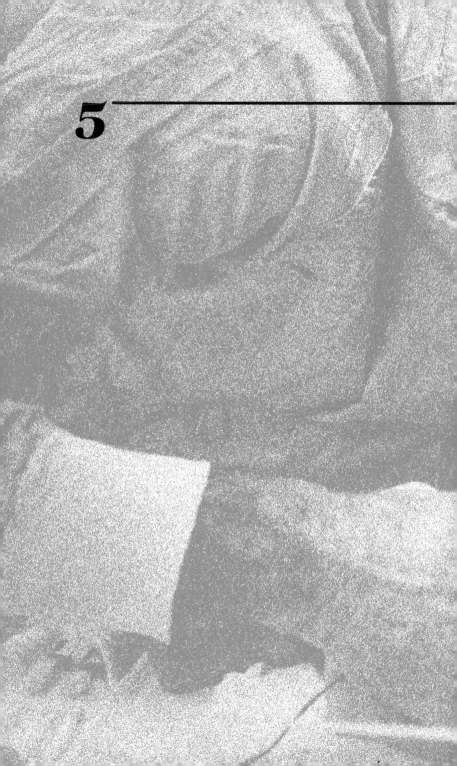

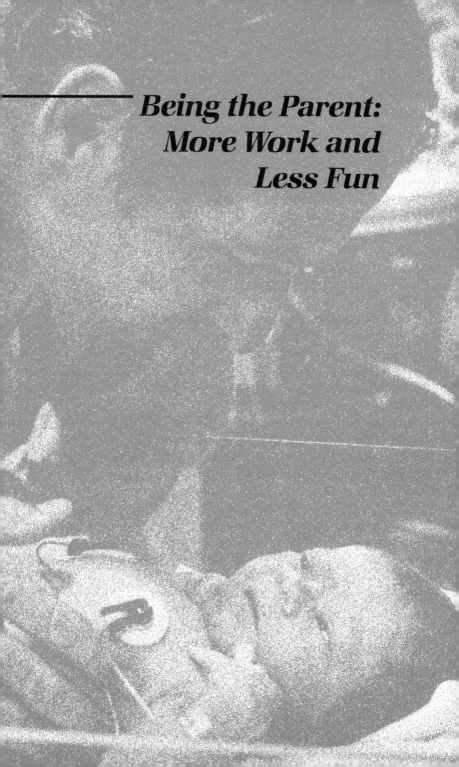

Being the Parent: More Work and Less Fun

Premature birth does more than bring a baby into the world before she is ready to be born. It also confers parenthood on two adults before they are ready and with more accompanying stress and anxiety than are usually expected. In our society, parenthood is associated with a mythology that makes it difficult and anxiety-producing even for parents of healthy full-term infants.

Currently popular views of child rearing convey the idea that the outcome of development is primarily attributable to parents' care and skill in raising children. When a child does well, parents take the credit for success. When a child fares badly, parents are expected to take the blame for failure. Given such overwhelming responsibility, many parents, especially with a first child, feel the pressure to do everything just right for fear that their child will be irreparably harmed by even small deviations from ideal care. In this atmosphere, each whimper or cry, each refused mouthful of food, or each skill that is mastered sooner by a neighbor's baby can become a sign that these parents must be doing something wrong. Fortunately, most parents soon realize that there is no ideal parent. If they have a second child or more, they discover that, even from the very first day, infants differ considerably from one another. It is easier to feel like a good parent with some babies than others.

However, caring for a premature infant adds numerous stresses and worries to the ordinary task of being a parent. In Chapter 4, we talked about some of the ways in which preterm babies are behaviorally and temperamentally more difficult to care for than their full-term counterparts. In this chapter, we talk about some of the other problems parents confront and discuss ways in which parents adapt to this difficult situation.

Besides having a baby who is easy to care for, what factors contribute to parents' skill and confidence? Most people who become parents for the first time have had many experiences in a variety of domains (work, family life, social life) that contribute to their general feeling of competence. When they begin to care for a new infant, they feel competent if they are able to readily interpret their baby's behavior, make quick and easy decisions about their own behavior, and find the baby responding in the way they expected or hoped. As they gain more experience with a particular baby, they are likely to become more skilled at interpreting the baby's behavior and making appropriate caregiving decisions. Feelings of self-confidence contribute to a parent's skill, for a parent who feels confident can make decisions easily and is not likely to be ruffled or upset by occasional disruptions. Such a parent is usually able to respond promptly and appropriately to the infant's behavior.

On the other hand, the parent who is lacking in

self-esteem finds it difficult to make decisions, feels unsure about whether she is doing the right thing, and may well communicate this sense of anxiety to the infant. Such a parent has difficulty in responding promptly and consistently to the infant's behavior. In the event of premature birth, most parents experience a series of damaging blows to their self-confidence before they have the opportunity to care for their baby.

Self-Confidence

Ingrid wept as she saw her daughter. "My third miscarriage," she said, just loud enough for those close to her to hear.[1]

At first, I was afraid to go to the nursery and see him. ... I didn't know what I would find. They practically had to drag me all the way the first time. [Mother at home visit 10 days after baby's discharge.][2]

I was really shocked. I was really tired out and I hadn't seen my baby and all I could think of was "My baby's very sick and they're going to take her away." I was really afraid she wasn't going to be with me very long. [Interview 1-month postdischarge.][3]

These are hardly the joyful responses we associate with the birth of a new baby. While it is true that the euphoria of new parenthood may be vastly overrated, we certainly would not expect grief, disappointment, shock, or fear—the feelings that these mothers of preterm infants expressed. These reactions are common ones to the event of premature birth. In fact, health-care professionals recognize the occurrence of a preterm birth as a family crisis.[4]

Usually a premature birth is unexpected:

We had just moved into a new apartment ... hadn't even unpacked when she went into labor.[5]

Our childbirth classes were supposed to start next week![6]

We were on vacation when my labor started. We had to go to a different hospital and I didn't even get my own doctor.[7]

These are the kinds of comments often heard when parents of preterm infants recount the experiences surrounding the births. In our own study sample, mothers who had given birth prematurely were more likely than those with term births to describe their experience as unpleasant or disappointing.[8] Ususally, the period of pregnancy is one of intense planning and preparation, and a premature birth invariably disrupts this process. It often entails the abandonment of plans in which parents have made intense emotional investments (for example, a relationship with an obstetrician, rooming in).

Many parents in this situation feel that they have failed to produce the normal, healthy infant they had fantasized, and they need to grieve for that infant before they can begin to form a relationship with the real-life baby they have.[9] Often, like Ingrid above, a woman delivers prematurely after a series of miscarriages and considers this birth yet another failure. Other mothers in the same situation may be enormously pleased to produce a live baby, however frail, after a series of unsuccessful pregnancies.

After the birth, parents confront numerous fears and anxieties about the health and welfare of their small, fragile baby. As we have seen in previous chapters, these worries have some realistic basis: the premature infant is more vulnerable to a variety of problems. With a baby who does have subsequent complications, parents may have to face the possibility that the infant will not survive and then, as the baby recovers, to adjust to his survival. There is also a certain amount of fear of attaching oneself to a loved one who may die, so that parents may feel ambivalent. Under these circumstances, it is difficult for parents to feel confident and enthusiastic about caring for their new infant. Each time they enter the nursery, they observe that a great deal of special equipment and training is necessary for the care of their infant, and they wonder how they will ever be able to manage on their own if and when the baby comes home. During this time, many parents express the feeling that they don't feel as if they have a baby; the baby seems to belong to the hospital.[10] With all these uncertainties, it is hard for the new mother of a preterm baby to feel competent.

One study asked mothers to choose either themselves or one of five other caregivers (father, nurse, doctor, experienced mother, grandmother) as the person best-suited to meet specific caregiving and socioemotional needs of infants.[11] Mothers with a first baby who was premature were unlikely to choose themselves if they had not been able to handle their infants in the nursery. Mothers of later-born infants were less affected by the opportunity to handle and care for their preterm infants. Presumably, they already had experiences that convinced them they were competent caregivers. However, the importance of opportunities to handle and care for infants during their hospitalization has been verified in a variety of ways.

Early Contact

In 1976, in a much-publicized book, Klaus and Kennell wrote:

> There is a sensitive period in the first minutes and hours of life during which it is necessary that the mother and father have close contact with their neonate for latter development to be optimal.[12]

Popular interpretations of such a statement tended to present an exaggerated tenet, which the authors later disowned as the "epoxy" theory of bonding.[13] This view assumes that there is a brief period immediately following birth when parents are malleable and capable of forming an emotional bond to their infant. After this period, the epoxy becomes fixed and, if the participants have been fortunate enough to have the "right" experience, they will be properly glued together or bonded. If they have been so unlucky as to have the "wrong" experience, they will be frozen in a separated or nonbonded state.

Recent reviews of the early-contact literature suggest that, while early contact does enhance parents' initial experiences and facilitate early parent–infant

relationships, there are few lasting effects.[14] Nevertheless, particularly when other circumstances militate
against a secure parent–infant relationship, early contact can make an important and beneficial contribution. Indeed, one of the main consequences of the
emphasis on early contact has been a major change
in hospital practices in the care of preterm infants.

Until the 1960s, nurseries caring for preterm infants
were preoccupied with maintaining a sterile environment to prevent the spread of infection. Parents were
looked on as simply another source of infection, and
their presence was to be minimized. Furthermore, it
was considered important to disturb these fragile babies
as little as possible, so that what parents might do
when they visited was even considered potentially
dangerous. Then a group at Stanford University Medical Center carried out what was, at the time, a very
daring experiment.[15] During part of the year, mothers
were encouraged to come to the nursery and handle
their preterm infants. Infection rates during these times
were compared with those during periods when parents were not allowed. The fact that there was no
increase in infection rate when parental visits were
allowed made possible the launching of a full-scale
study of the effects of early contact versus separation
in the premature nursery. A similar study was begun
in Cleveland at Case Western Reserve Medical Center.[16]

We have already mentioned one finding from the
Stanford study: the mothers who were allowed into
the nursery were more self-confident than those who
were not. They were also, at first, more skillful in handling their babies. By one month after the baby's discharge, these differences were no longer evident. At

the first pediatric checkup, there were no differences between the two groups in maternal behavior, though both differed from a comparison group of full-term mothers in smiling less at their infants and making less body contact with them.[17]

In the Cleveland study, mothers in the contact group spent more time face to face with their infants and more time cuddling them than did mothers in the separated group.[18] Although there were some later differences reported in infant skills, there were few differences in maternal behavior that could be attributed to the early contact experience. Nevertheless, the benefits to mothers, even short-term were important, and the findings from these studies have played a major role in changing hospital procedures in preterm nurseries. Currently, the majority of hospitals allow both mothers and fathers to visit, and most also invest time and effort in helping parents to cope with the stressful experiences surrounding the birth and care of their infants. Mothers, for example, are often encouraged to breast-feed their preterm infants and are shown how to express and save breast milk for their infant's early tube or bottle feedings until nursing is possible.[19] Fathers are encouraged to visit the nursery and, especially when mothers are themselves hospitalized, to bring back pictures and news of the baby to share (Figure 1). In fact, it has often been noted that fathers of preterm infants are sometimes more involved with their care than are fathers of full-term newborns.[20] This may be a consequence of the special role they had to play during the early weeks after the infant's birth.

Even with these changes, the early experiences of parents with their preterm baby are still quite different

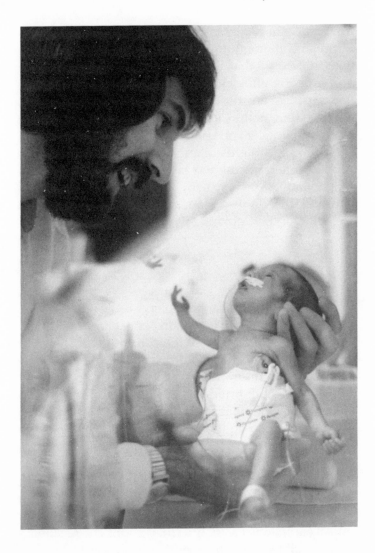

Figure 1 *A father interacting with his preterm baby in the isolette.*
[Photograph copyright © Bob Stewart.]

from those of parents who take home a healthy, full-term baby after a 3- to 5-day hospital stay. Often, parents are advised that, once the preterm infant is healthy and growing, they can now go home and treat their baby just like any other healthy baby. Yet, as we know from Chapter 4, the baby they are taking home may be temperamentally and behaviorally quite different from the average full-term infant. Thus, parents of premature infants have many reasons to feel anxious and inadequate, and their baby is likely to be difficult to care for. How do they manage? Most of the time, quite well. Sometimes, quite badly.

Caretaking Casualty

The term "caretaking casualty" is used to describe a range of inadequate caretaking situations, including, at the most extreme end of the continuum, abuse and neglect.[21] Several studies of the developmental characteristics of children included in abuse and neglect statistics have reported that 20–40% of the study sample were born prematurely.[22] Since only 5–7% of births are premature, even the low figure of 20% exceeds the expected occurrence of preterm births among victims of failures in parenting. When the idea of a sensitive period was first introduced, the long parent–infant separation endured during the infant's hospitalization was considered to be a possible reason for the high rate of caretaking casualty in this group. The reasoning was as follows: When parents are unable to be with their infant during this very important early sensitive period, they are denied the opportunity to form an appropriate relationship with their infants at the optimal time. They must then form their emotional ties to the infant at a later time, when it is more difficult, and this leads to a higher rate of failure.

However, recent observational studies of parents with their preterm infant suggest that early separation may not be the most important factor affecting parent relationships with preterm infants. One study compared three groups of infants and their parents: (1) preterm infants who had experienced respiratory distress and had been hospitalized prior to discharge, (2) postterm infants who had been treated like normal infants in the normal nursery but, like the preterm infants, had obtained poor scores on the Brazelton scales, indicating that they were behaviorally difficult, and (3) healthy, full-term infants.[23] Patterns of parent behavior were similar in the preterm and postterm groups, even though they were dissimilar in amount of early contact, and both differed from the parents of full-term infants.

In a review of studies of parent–infant interaction that included preterm infants, the data were quite similar, in spite of drawing on births in six different hospitals where the amount of early contact between parents and infants varied considerably—from none to daily visiting.[24] Finally, in one of the most direct studies of early contact at Stanford Medical Center, while the contact and separation groups did show early differences, by four months postdischarge, they were similar to each other, though both differed from the full-term comparison group.[25] On the other hand, a study of maternal visiting patterns showed that mothers who had little contact with their hospitalized infants (less than 3 visits per two weeks) were more likely to abandon them, give them up for adoption, or care for them inadequately than mothers who visited more often.[26] How can we reconcile these conflicting findings?

What seems a most likely explanation is that all of the stressful conditions we have already discussed combine to place the preterm infant at risk for care-taking casualty. Separation is only one contributing condition. A difficult and unrewarding baby is another. The anxieties and problems surrounding the parents' experience of the birth and care of the preterm infant are a third group of contributing factors. Finally, we should bear in mind the point made in the Introduction that a good number of preterm infants are born to families already experiencing economic, social, and/or medical problems. When many of these stresses are simultaneously present and parents do not have adequate support from family, friends, or professionals, a failure in child care is more likely to occur. In the vast majority of cases, this does not happen. What about the remaining families with preterm infants?

Parent–Infant Interaction

In the 1970s, with the knowledge that preterm infants were at risk for caretaking casualties, a number of studies comparing parent–infant interaction with preterm and full-term infants were begun. One rationale of many of these studies was that pathological patterns of parental behavior were more likely to be observed in the preterm groups, and the identification of differences between full-term and preterm groups would give us tools for the identification of parents with problems. Most of these studies did indeed find differences between preterm and full-term interactions. However, they were not always consistent with the predictions made, and it has become clear that it may be very difficult to decide what is pathological and what is adaptive coping behavior of parents.

A common finding by researchers who observed parents and infants in the newborn period was that parents of preterm infants were less actively engaged with their baby than were the parents of full-term babies. They were likely to hold the baby farther away, talk to the baby less, make fewer attempts at face-to-face contact, and do less affectionate touching.[27] These data were usually interpreted as indicative of difficulties that parents of preterm infants experienced in becoming attached to their babies.

When we planned our own longitudinal study, we expected that this was a pattern that would continue as we followed parents and infants over the first year of life. However, when we looked at data from our observations at 4, 8, and 12 months, we were quite surprised to find that our predictions were wrong. At 4 months, the differences we had seen in newborn feedings were still there, but greatly diminished.[28] At 8 months, during floor-play observations, we noted that parents of preterm infants who had experienced respiratory distress were more active than those of full-term infants rather than less.[29] They stayed closer to their babies, touched them more, and offered and demonstrated toys more often. The only thing they did less of was smiling, and that was not surprising because their infants played with toys less and fussed more

than their full-term peers. By 12 months, there were
no differences between groups in patterns of interaction during floor play.

As we began to review other studies, it became
clear that this was a common finding in studies where
the infants were beyond the newborn period: where
there were differences, parents of preterm infants were
more active than their full-term counterparts rather
than less. For example, one study reported that, within
the preterm group, babies who had experienced more
early medical problems subsequently received more
caregiving from their parents than did their healthier
peers.[30] Another study found that at feedings 1 and 3
months postdischarge, mothers of preterm infants were
more active than those in the full-term group, while
their babies were less active participants than were the
full-term infants.[31] The same pattern was observed in
a very different task.[32] Mothers were asked to try to
interest their 11-month-olds in some new play materials—a cup and some blocks. The full-term infants
were more likely than the preterm infants to play independently with the materials, but the mothers of the
preterm infants spent more time actively involved with
the task than did their full-term counterparts.

In the study by Field discussed earlier, mothers
were asked to engage in face-to-face play with their
3½-month-old babies.[33] The mothers in the preterm
group were more active than those in the full-term
group, while their infants were less attentive and more
fussy than the full-term group. In both groups, when
mothers were asked to imitate their babies, they engaged
in less activity and their babies became more attentive.
From Chapter 3, you may recall that preterm infants

often seem to be inefficient information processors, and it has been suggested that their frequent inattention is a way of avoiding an information overload. When the mother's activity exceeds an infant's ability to process information, he turns away. When mothers present smaller amounts of information at a slower rate, babies do not need to turn away as often.

On the other hand, we also noted in Chapter 3 that preterm infants, at least when young, have a high threshold for some kinds of stimulation. That is, they need more or stronger stimulation before they respond to sound and touch. When parents try to adjust to this high threshold, they probably do so by increasing their efforts to elicit a response. If this interpretation is correct, it is easy to see how difficult it is for the parent of a preterm infant to avoid a frustrating cycle. The baby needs a lot of stimulation but, when the parent tries to provide it, the baby becomes overloaded and must take time out by turning away. So the more the parent works, the less the infant may attend. As one mother of an 8-month-old preterm boy said,

> I think he needs a lot of stimulation. I know I sometimes overdo it but if I don't keep him going, he'll just lie there and do nothing. I figure it's better to give him too much than to let him vegetate.[34]

Thus, while the high activity rate of parents with their preterm infants sometimes seems maladaptive to observers, it may be the best compromise under the circumstances.

As we noted earlier, in our own study, most differences between preterm and full-term groups in interaction style have disappeared by 12 months of age. A preliminary report from a study of mothers and toddlers 9–24 months old repeats this pattern.[35] Mothers of preterm infants at 9 months were more active than those of full-term infants in such areas as physical and verbal teaching and expressed concern with infant needs and intentions. By 12 months, these differences were no longer apparent. The authors of this study interpret the findings as follows. The mothers of preterm infants are engaged in a self-designed intervention program to provide extra stimulation to the babies that they perceive as developmentally delayed in cognitive and motor skills. By the end of the first year, when most preterm babies appear to have "caught up" with their postnatal age mates, mothers judge that their stimulation program has been successful and is no longer necessary.

Pathology and Adaptation

Although many of the studies discussed above were designed to identify pathology in the social interactions of parents and their preterm infants, it is difficult to characterize the behaviors described as pathological. Stressful, often unrewarding, less fun than those of their full-term counterparts—yes. But since they occur so frequently among parents with preterm infants across different situations and study samples, it appears that we are observing what is "normal" for parents of preterm infants. It is normal for parents of preterm infants to take a longer time to become actively involved in social interactions with their babies. It is normal for these same parents to work harder for less reward. Moreover, this seems to be a common parental adaptation to some other developmental problems as well.[36] We must remember that the majority of these infants do develop normally and are not mistreated by their parents. In many of these studies, most of the differences between preterm and full-term groups disappear toward the end of the first year. These parents must be doing something right—with much difficulty and stress, but probably basically right.

Our hunch about what is happening is based on a description of the developing parent–infant relationship as a series of adjustments that parents must make as their babies grow, develop, and change.[37] Each time the baby acquires new skills, parents must adjust accordingly, and each new stage of infant development requires renegotiation of the rules of interaction. At first, the major issue is the infant's physiological functioning and the need to establish routines of eating and sleeping. Later, when the baby becomes more alert and socially responsive, the challenge is to establish mutually enjoyable social games. Still later, the infant's ability to take the initiative and to assert independence provides other occasions to establish new interaction patterns.

It may be that, for prematurely born infants and their parents, the adjustment to each new stage is more difficult and on the average takes longer than for full-term infants and their parents. However, the majority of parent–infant pairs do eventually make a moderately successful adjustment to each new stage. Because the preterm infant is often behaviorally and temperamentally different from the typical full-term infant of the same developmental age, what is appropriate for preterm interactions may look different from what is adaptive in full-term interactions.

There are several ways in which most parents rise to the challenges of caring for a prematurely born infant. First, they invest more time and effort than they would with a full-term infant. Second, they develop patterns and styles of interaction that differ in some respects from those parents with a full-term infant. In addition, they often depend on extended family, friends, or health-care professionals for support. We have already noted that fathers often become more involved in the care of a preterm infant than they might with a full-term baby. In our own study, we observed that, in addition to meeting more of the fathers in the preterm group, we also met other relatives and friends more often than in the full-term group. Thus, a supporting network of family and friends, as well as health-care professionals, seems to be especially important to the parents of infants born prematurely.

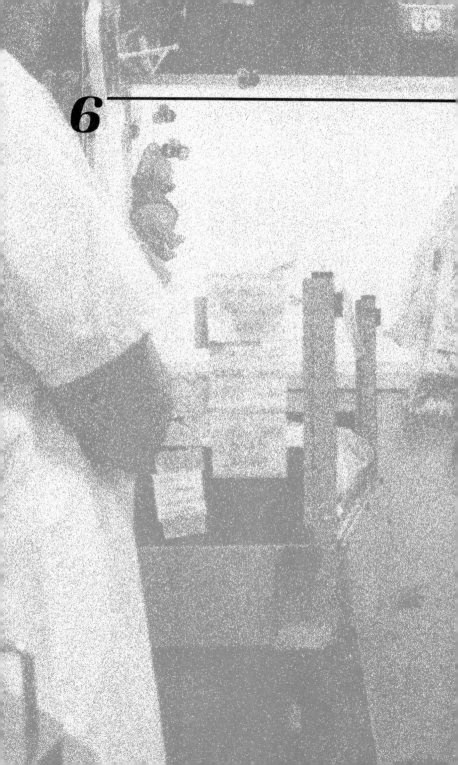

6

Intervention Programs: Support for Infant and Parent

Since the prematurely born infant is more vulnerable than the average full-term infant to developmental difficulties and is likely to make heavier demands on parents' skills and patience, what can be done to prevent or ameliorate these problems? Many experimental studies have asked whether specific experiences during or after intensive care have improved the health or behavioral development of preterm infants. In this chapter, we discuss the reasoning behind such intervention programs, look at some examples, and summarize the findings.

In addition to experimental programs, there are also numerous hospitals, clinics, and private practitioners caring for preterm infants and their parents on an individual clinical basis. These treatments designed for the well-being of a particular infant and family cannot be evaluated systematically. However, some of the strategies and techniques used in these settings will be mentioned. It is important to bear in mind that, for any particular baby and family, such individual care, tailored to the needs, temperaments, and skills in each case, is likely to be more beneficial than any standard program routinely administered to large numbers of infants and families. When an experimental treatment in a systematic study is found to have beneficial effects, it usually means that it was a good match for many of the babies or families studied. It does not necessarily mean that every single case in the experimental group benefited or showed equally dramatic gains.

With this in mind, we consider two general kinds of interventions: those carried out in the hospital before discharge, and those designed to assist babies and families after hospital discharge. Some programs include both types of intervention. Most programs of the first kind focus exclusively on stimulation of the infant alone, although, as we will see, such programs can also have effects on parents. Among the few programs designed to follow preterm infants after discharge, some focus primarily on the infant, but all involve parent stimulation of the infant and some include additional help for parents.

Experimental programs to foster development of preterm infants in the hospital have often assumed that the intensive-care unit is a stimulus-deprivation condition, pointing to the unchanging temperature and illumination levels, minimal movement, and lack of social interaction as evidence. But as we saw in Chapter 1, intensive-care units can, in many respects, be considered conditions of overstimulation. The illumination and noise levels are high, and the number and frequency of nursing and medical interventions may also be high. (Recall, for example, that, in one hospital, an infant might be cared for by 70 different nurses during a stay in intensive care.)

An intervention strategy that has not been used

is one that tries to minimize potentially aversive experiences by muffling noise, periodically dimming lights to simulate night and day, or varying the pattern and frequency of necessary nursing and medical care. Many questions can be raised in conjunction with this strategy:

> Is it better to disturb a baby fewer times and carry out several uncomfortable procedures at the same time or to disturb the baby more often and allow recovery each time?

> How often is it really necessary to draw blood, take temperature, and change sheets?

> Are the benefits in medical and nursing care worth the possible physiological or psychological costs to the baby?

Sometimes complicated technology leads us to forget that there may be less intrusive methods of getting information. Behavioral observations can sometimes supplement or substitute for more disturbing methods, such as taking repeated blood samples. This is not to suggest that blood samples should not be drawn, but only that they might, in some cases, be drawn less often, without loss of information if the infant's appearance and behavior are monitored more carefully. As we indicated in Chapter 1, routines in intensive-care units are not intended to benefit psychosocial and behavioral development; these are considered luxuries during medical crises. Nevertheless, now that we have the technology to manage physical care, it is time to ask whether the psychological quality of intensive care can be improved. Figure 1 shows a

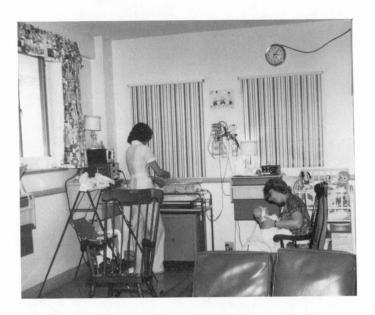

Figure 1   *The Family Care Center, The Children's Hospital, Denver, Colorado. [Photograph courtesy of Edward Goldson, M.D.]*

unit in which infants who are no longer acutely ill, but still require a great deal of nursing care may have a more pleasant experience than the typical preterm units provides.

Several experimental studies have asked whether the provision of special experiences during intensive care can improve the health and behavioral development of preterm babies. The reasoning behind these interventions is usually based on one of two ideas: the first is that the preterm infant is really an extrauterine fetus, while the second assumes that preterm babies are small, immature newborns.

Simulating the Womb During Hospitalization

Interventions based on the first approach have tried to make the experience of the preterm in intensive care more womblike. Most often, such interventions focus on the fact that, before birth, the baby experiences a variety of movements as the mother carries out her daily activities, while the typical incubator is stationary. Various techniques have been devised to provide more movement for preterm infants. For example, a motorized hammock was designed to rotate and swing the infant in a rhythmic fashion.[1] From the fifth day after birth until they reached a postconception age of 36 weeks, 31 babies were placed in the hammock three times daily for 30 minutes. When compared with 31 babies who did not get this experience, the stimulated babies had gained more weight and performed better on the Graham–Rosenblith scales, especially on motor skills and responses to visual and auditory stimulation.

A different technique for providing movement was a rocker that was automatically turned on for 15 minutes every hour.[2] In addition, in order to reproduce some of the sounds a baby might hear before birth, tape recordings of heartbeats were played during the periods of rocking: 7 infants were exposed to this treatment for two weeks 33 and 34 weeks postconception. To see whether this treatment was effective, the investigator examined weight gain, neurological maturation, and wake–sleep patterns. As infants mature, waking and sleeping alternate more regularly, and the amount of time spent in deep or quiet sleep increases, while the time spent in light or active sleep decreases. Infants in the study were observed three times weekly for 2½ hours on each occasion to record wake–sleep patterns. In comparison to the 8 control babies, the experimental infants showed more mature wake–sleep patterns. They spent more time in quiet sleep and less in active sleep. Although the differences were not great, the stimulated infants also gained more weight and showed more rapid neurological maturation.

More recently, in attempts to approximate the fluid environment of the uterus, preterm infants have been placed on waterbeds. In one study, the waterbed was constantly rocked mechanically.[3] Although the 10 infants in the waterbeds did not differ from the 11 controls in weight gain, vital signs, or how often they spit up feedings, they were less likely to have interruptions in breathing. A later study using the waterbed rocked the infants for 1 hour before each feeding, while tapes of a heartbeat and a woman's voice were played.[4] The 11 infants in the stimulated group gained more weight and grew more (as measured by head circumference) than the 9 controls. There were no differences between the groups in neurological maturation or behavior skills demonstrated on the Brazelton assessment.

Simulating the Home During Hospitalization

An entirely different approach to the appropriate environment for preterm infants assumes that "normal" experience is not that of the womb, but that of infants in the full-term nursery and in their homes.

The preterm infant, according to this view, is being deprived of the experience of being held, touched, and carried, of seeing people and toys, and of hearing human voices. Interventions based on this reasoning include hanging mobiles over cribs, playing tape-recorded voices and, most often, handling the infant regularly in a soothing or playful manner.

One of the first studies of this kind assigned preterm infants to either high or low handling conditions.[5] In the high condition, beginning 7–10 days after birth, infants received 260 minutes of stroking, rocking, and holding on each of 14 consecutive days (Figure 2). Over the same period of time, the low handling group received 95 minutes per day of similar experience. Although there were no differences between groups in weight gain, the babies who received extra handling spent more time in quiet states. Other studies that provided extra handling of this type for preterm infants have reported weight gains[6] although sometimes only temporary ones,[7] more efficient feeding,[8] and superior performance on the Brazelton scales.[9]

A second example of this type of study involved more extensive additions to the preterm infants' experiences. Mobiles were hung for infants to look at, nurses provided regular play periods during which they rocked, patted, and talked to the babies, and nurses held the babies close during feedings so that the baby could see the nurse's face.[10] Before these changes were introduced, the 15 controls were slightly superior to the 15 experimental infants in behavior skills as assessed by the Brazelton scales. After 4 weeks of the experimental treatment, the stimulated infants had gained more weight and showed superior performance on the Brazelton scales.

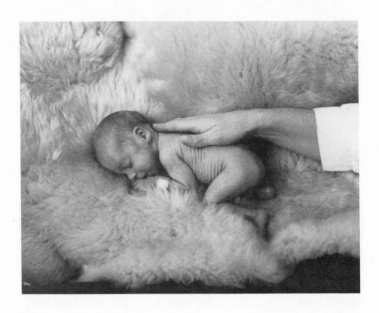

Figure 2 *A preterm infant being gently stroked while lying on a soft lamb's-wool rug. [Photograph copyright © Suzanne Arms/Jeroboam, Inc.]*

In all of these studies attempting to make the intensive-care unit more homelike, the experimental handling was carried out by nurses or research staff. We have already mentioned, in the Introduction and in Chapter 5, that opportunities to handle and care for their infants in intensive care are important to parents. One study tried to find out whether the same kind of handling administered by nurses and mothers might have different effects.[11] Perhaps when the mother herself does the handling, there are benefits to the mother–infant relationship that can further enhance the infant's development. In this study, the 24 infants who were handled (13 by nurses, 11 by mothers) regained their birthweight faster than the 8 controls, but there were no differences between the mother-handled and nurse-handled groups either in the hospital or at later follow-ups. One possible reason that handling by mothers was not more effective was that the mothers in this group varied widely in the frequency of their visits. The average rate of visiting was only once every 4 days (in contrast to the nurses' daily stimulation). However, with this in mind, it is tempting to suggest that the mothers were indeed more effective since they accomplished as much as the nurses in fewer episodes of contact.

With the exception of this study, none of the above reports asked how parents might be affected by infant stimulation. However, one of the benefits of supplemental stimulation programs might be to provide parents with an infant who is more responsive and rewarding, thus enhancing the care the infant receives after discharge. One of the most intriguing studies of early stimulation suggests that effects on parent behavior can be found even during the infant's hospitalization.[12] The babies in this study, 48 preterm infants, were divided into two groups: 24 who were given two daily 20-minute periods of exercises by a nurse–technician, and 24 controls who were given routine treatment. Parents in both groups knew that their babies were to be followed after discharge. Parents of infants in the experimental group knew that their babies were being exercised regularly and that they would be shown some exercises to do with the baby after discharge. Both groups of parents were allowed to visit as much as they wished. During the infant's hospitalization, 92%

of the parents in the intervention group visited at least once, while only 62% of the control infants were visited. Furthermore, of those visited, parents whose babies were in the intervention group visited on the average 4–5 times weekly during the first half of the infant's hospital stay, while the parents of control infants visited 2½–3 times weekly in the same period. These differences were not explainable by differences in parent educational levels, income, parity, marital status, or distance from the hospital.

However, there was some indication that the babies in the experimental group became more alert than their controls. This suggests that parents in the intervention group might have visited more often because they found their babies more alert and therefore more fun to visit than were the babies in the control group. It is also possible that parents in the experimental group thought about their babies differently because they knew they were getting special treatment. This study does point out that many of the programs we have been discussing may have had similar, though unmeasured effects on the parents of the infants.

Meeting Parental Needs During Hospitalization

As we have pointed out, parents of preterm infants have many problems of their own during the hospitalization of their baby. They are worried and anxious about the baby and are trying to cope with complicated medical information and terminology. They may also feel guilty, depressed, or angry at the differences between the experiences they expected and those that actually confront them. How can parents be helped during this stressful time? In many intensive-care units, the nurses are trained to attend as best they can to parent needs for attention, care, and assistance. In most units, one or more social workers are also available and responsible for the care of parents, while nurses and doctors care for the babies. In some instances, efforts have been made to have "veteran" parents of preterm infants share their experiences with new parents in individual or group meetings.

We know of only one attempt to evaluate such a program. At the Hospital for Sick Children in Toronto, a study was conducted of 28 families of sick preterm infants.[13] The parents had met weekly for 7–12 weeks in small groups with a veteran parent and a nurse coordinator. The control group was 29 families of similar background whose infants were also small, sick, and born prematurely. Some of the group meetings were concerned with sharing feelings of distress; others provided information about the care of preterm infants through the use of slides, films, and other informational aids. The nurse coordinator was also available to help individual parents with specific problems of their own such as finding baby-sitters or collecting unemployment benefits.

The mothers who participated in the group sessions visited their infants more often and were more active with their infants during visits than were the mothers in the comparison group. At the time of the babies' discharge, ratings based on interviews with the mothers revealed that those who had attended group meetings were more likely to be satisfied with the medical and nursing care of their baby, to have a better understanding of their infant's problems, to be more confident about their ability to care for the baby at home, and to be more familiar with community resources than were those who had not had the opportunity for group experiences. Thus, it seems that the opportunity to meet with other parents who have had similar experiences and problems is helpful during the infant's hospitalization.

On the basis of increased understanding of the problems of preterm infants and their parents, more and more hospitals are trying to make special-care units as comfortable as possible for babies and their parents. Parents may be encouraged to decorate their baby's area in the nursery, to bring toys, pictures, mobiles, and baby clothes from home. The furnishings may include comfortable chairs, and there may be reading materials for parents. In recognition of the needs of new families, some units include rooms where parents may live with their baby before his discharge and where siblings and other relatives may visit. In addition, efforts of nurses, social workers, or parent groups may be directed toward helping parents to enjoy their baby as well as to understand and accept their problems as parents of a special baby.

Programs After Discharge

Most of the intensive efforts to enhance the health and development of preterm infants are focused on the hospital period. During this time, babies and families are in contact with hospital workers, and equipment for special stimulation or testing is more likely to be available. Once babies are discharged, their families are dispersed over a wide geographic area, and the ease with which special programs can be carried out depends on how readily families can visit the hospital or be visited at home. A regional special-care unit may serve several states, so that some families lose contact with hospital staff once their babies go home. For this reason, it is more difficult to design and carry out programs for continuing intervention, and there are fewer examples of this type of program. Many parents who were glowing and enthusiastic in their praise of the help and support received during the infant's hospitalization feel "abandoned" once they take their baby home.

In our own study, we visited families at home 10 days after the baby's discharge.[14] Although our main purpose was to collect information, we found that families were eager to see us and had "saved up" many practical questions to ask us that they deemed "not important enough to bother my pediatrician." We were asked what we thought about pacifiers, how long to breast-feed on each side, whether babies could be spoiled by too much attention, and so on. Thus, many families in our research project considered us resource people and felt supported by our regular visits and discussions. One mother enrolled her second child, a healthy, full-term boy, in a later longitudinal project and remarked to us how wonderful such projects were.

> After all, who else will come and visit you in the middle of the winter when you're stuck at home with a small baby? Who else will listen to you talk about your baby for a whole hour without getting bored?[15]

Thus, many families with young infants, especially those born prematurely, are eager for continued attention from health-care professionals long after their babies have left the hospital.

One program that provided such attention was part of a study of in-hospital treatment as well.[16] Earlier, we mentioned that extra attention was given to the experimental babies in this study during their hospital stay. Later on, the families in the experimental group were visited weekly by a social worker. The home visitor pointed out activities to encourage specific skills (for example, dangling toys for babies starting to reach for things, playing patty-cake for those starting to use both hands together). Toys were provided for some of these activities, and the home visitor was also available to help the mother with her own questions, worries, and needs. At 1 year of age, the infants in this group were performing at expected age level on developmental tests, while the control infants were lagging behind. Since the babies in the experimental group were treated differently both in the hospital and at home, it is difficult to know how much each part of the intervention program contributed to their age-appropriate development. Nevertheless, this study demonstrates that, with appropriate intervention and support, most preterm babies—even in disadvantaged families, such as were in this sample—can develop normally.

One short-term study that began after hospital discharge involved teaching mothers a special massage and rocking procedure.[17] This was carried out four times each day for a month, with the help of regular visits from a nurse. When they were 4 months of age, the 15 infants who received this treatment were neurologically more mature, had gained more weight, and performed better on the Bayley scales than did the 14 controls.

A more ambitious study attempted to provide individualized intervention programs to 30 families of preterm infants who were part of a larger follow-up study.[18] From the time the infants were 10 months old until they were 2, they were visited by project staff members who tried to help mothers interact with their baby in ways that matched each infant's skills and temperament. For each family, an individualized plan was designed on the basis of prior information from the follow-up study and from initial visits by the staff of the intervention program. The progress of the infants, as well as the development of the parent–child relationship, was compared with that of other families in the follow-up program with similar characteristics. Data from home observations at 24 months indicated that parents in the intervention group were more likely to provide appropriate activities for their infants and were more sensitive observers of their babies than were those in the control group. Thus, the intervention did seem to foster parent–child interaction. However, it was expected that more effective parent–child interaction would also be associated with superior cognitive skills. This expectation was not borne out. The failure to find differences in cognitive performance may reflect the fact that both groups had free medical and nursing care through the infant's second birthday, including postdischarge visits by nurses, support from social workers, and regular follow-up assessments with referrals for special problems. Thus, both groups were extensively supported through the child's early years.

This particular program illustrates the kind of follow-up supports and services that might be routinely available to families after their infant's discharge. Many hospitals do have follow-up clinics to monitor the development of preterm infants and to make referrals for special treatment when necessary. However, it is unusual for medical, nursing, and follow-up services to be provided without financial cost to parents, and it is equally unusual for all infants to be routinely included in such arrangements. More often, a smaller group of families, those who can get to the hospital easily, who have adequate medical coverage, and who are aggressive in seeking out resources, are able to make use of such facilities. Alternatively, hospitals may aggressively seek out, follow, and support families whose infants are of special concern. This may include infants who had serious or multiple problems or who are receiving a particular medical treatment. In many cities, parent self-help organizations have begun support groups where parents can share the experience of caring for preterm infants.

Throughout this book, we have tried to emphasize that what is normal or optimal for the preterm infant, particularly the small, sick preterm baby, may be quite different from what is optimal for the full-term baby. Similarly, the goal in intervention programs need not be to make the experience of preterm infants more like that of full-term infants, but to make it more appropriate to their special needs. For example, when feeding a full-term newborn, we consider it desirable to hold the baby close, try to make eye contact, and provide some affectionate social experience. For the small, sick preterm, all of this might be too much at once.

These babies may turn away, gag, or develop breathing difficulties during an overstimulating feeding.

A dramatic example of this was an infant who was quite small and ill and was feeding poorly.[19] The only nurse in the unit who was able to feed this baby successfully was the one who admitted disliking the infant intensely. The secret of her success was that she interacted with him as little as possible during feedings. This may seem "abnormal" or "disturbed" when compared with typical feedings of full-term babies; yet for this small, fragile infant, feedings went best when he had to cope only with the bottle rather than with the bottle plus a sociable person. Of course, this would not be the case for every preterm baby, especially after several months at home.

This example highlights the importance of treating each baby as an individual. The purpose of all the experiments described in this chapter was to demonstrate various techniques and programs of stimulation that might be useful in enhancing the development of preterm infants and their interaction with their parents. In most cases, the decision to use any of these procedures with a particular baby or family rests appropriately with the attending physician, the family, and, as the above example demonstrates, the infant. When an infant tries to tell us that he is not benefiting from a particular treatment, adult caregivers bear the responsibility for taking that message seriously and acting on it.

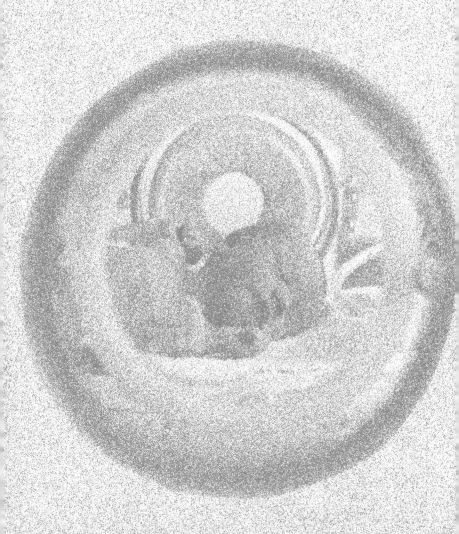

Summary:
Putting It All
Together

We began this book with the idea that, if we summarized what is known about the development of children born prematurely, we would be able to answer some important questions, not only about the effects of prematurity, but also about the nature of development. In this concluding chapter, we will see what kinds of answers we can give to those questions. In addition, we will highlight some of the recurrent themes that have been mentioned only briefly in previous chapters.

One such theme is the difficulty of isolating effects attributable to prematurity alone, as opposed to those associated with prior or subsequent conditions surrounding premature birth. We noted in the Introduction that, about half the time, it is possible to identify conditions likely to have caused a premature birth. These conditions involve physical, social, or psychological stresses to the mother and family that in themselves may handicap a child's development. In Chapter 1, we noted that many of the infants born prematurely encounter subsequent medical problems resulting directly or indirectly from physiological immaturity. In these cases, both the medical problems and the treatments they require can have residual effects on development.

Additionally, several questions have been raised about the early psychological and social experiences of infants who spend long periods of time in intensive-care units. This is a relatively new concern because it was only after most of the medical and technical aspects of preterm care had been mastered that the concern for psychological well-being could be addressed. Thus, this is still a controversial area, with inadequate information and many differing opinions about effects on development.

In Chapters 4 and 5, we noted that, for both the infant and the parent, the stresses associated with preterm birth make it difficult to establish an optimal parent–child relationship and that this difficulty can persist well into the first year. How much longer it persists is not yet known. Nevertheless, since infants are dependent upon adult care for survival and since the preterm infant is in even more need of good care than is the average infant, difficulties in parent–infant interaction add yet another risk factor to the developmental process. With such a litany of disadvantages, the most surprising finding is that the majority of preterm infants do not fulfill what might be considered a prophecy of doom. In fact, most develop normally. In the concluding section of the chapter, we return to this finding, which is probably the most important and striking of those we have discussed. Our concern here is whether we can isolate the separate effects of each of these potentially contributing factors to the developmental process.

What makes it difficult to identify specific effects of premature birth or of other stressful conditions surrounding it is that the conditions do not occur independently. Instead, they tend to occur together and to vary together. That is, mothers living under the most stressful and inadequate conditions have the greatest chance of giving birth to the young, small infants who are most vulnerable to complications. It is these same fragile babies who spend the longest time in the hospital, creating the most stressful circumstances for the parent–infant relationship. Subsequently, these infants, who are most in need of good physical and psychological care, are discharged to the inadequate home environment that may have caused their early birth in the first place. Under these circumstances, how do we know whether poor developmental progress reflects the prematurity of birth, damage from medical complications, or inadequate care after hospital discharge?

The ideal study to answer these questions would compare babies who are similar in every respect except the one we wish to study—say, age at birth. So we would want to select several groups of babies born at different gestational ages. One group might be 36- and 37-week-olds, another 34- and 35-week-olds, still another 32- and 33-week-olds, and so on. You can see that, as soon as we tried to match these groups for birthweight, we would be in trouble. The younger babies would invariably be those with lower birthweights, and the older babies with very low birthweights would be small for their age, adding an unwanted complication to the study design. But, in the ideal experiment, we would want to match our groups on many other factors besides birthweight: maternal health history, type and severity of infant complications, length of hospital stay, and the like. Obviously, this ideal study (like most ideal studies) could not possibly be done.

An alternative strategy is to use statistical methods to compute estimates of how much each factor of interest contributes to a particular outcome. As we pointed out in Chapter 2, this is the approach that most recent studies have used. However, what is important to us here is that what may seem at first glance to be technicalities of research design really tell us something about the nature of the developmental process.

The attempt to isolate simple cause-and-effect relationships in development is based on the idea that a specific event at one time (for example, birth at 34 weeks of gestation) should have a specific and measurable effect on outcome at a later time (for example, IQ score at age 5). This approach requires the assumption that all events occurring between these two points of interest are irrelevant or have, at most, negligible relationships with the early (potentially causal) event and the later measures. A simple cause-and-effect model of this sort is represented in Figure 1. It would be very convenient if a simple model such as this were generally useful, but in real life there are very few instances where such a straightforward relationship holds.

In real life, birth at 34 weeks' gestational age would be accompanied by many other events—some related to the premature birth, others not. Similarly, many aspects of experience will influence IQ score at age 5— some related to the preterm birth, others not. In order to estimate the effects of preterm birth on later IQ scores,

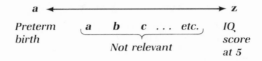

Figure 1 *Simple prediction from early event to outcome.*

it is necessary to have some idea of how the intervening events are related to both the initial event and the outcome in our prediction problem.

One kind of relationship would be that of a chain of short-term "causes" that link the two endpoints. Such a chain is illustrated in Figure 2. Here, rather than asking how event *a* (birth at 34 weeks' gestational age) is directly related to *z* (IQ score at age 5), we try to trace the effect of *a* on *b* (which might represent the presence or absence of respiratory distress), the relationship of *b* to *c* (which might be the length of the hospital stay), the effect of *c* on *d* (which might be parental attitudes), and so on. Here we do not expect to predict *z* from *a* alone, but from *a* in conjunction with *b*, *c*, *d*, and so on. Thus, a preterm birth leads to certain early experiences for both parents and infants that establish conditions for caregiving at home. Early caregiving influences development in the first weeks of life, which in turn affects parental attitudes and caregiving practices, and so on.

Even this kind of causal chain, which is considerably more complex than the simple cause-and-effect model, is probably far too simple for real life. For example, Figure 3 illustrates a model in which each link in

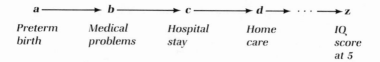

Preterm   Medical   Hospital   Home   IQ
birth   problems   stay   care   score
                                             at 5

Figure 2   *Prediction from early event to outcome through a chain of intervening events.*

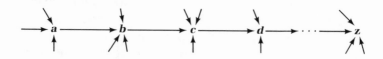

Figure 3   *Prediction via a chain of events taking account of multiple influences at all points.*

the causal chain is viewed as a consequence of multiple causes. Thus, preterm birth is surrounded by many conditions that contribute to the infant's physical and developmental status at discharge. Caregiving at home will be affected by the infant's condition at discharge plus factors such as family size, life style, and access to medical care and social services.

To complicate our view of development even more, notice that, in all of the figures so far, all of the arrows suggest influence in one direction only. But as we have noted earlier in this chapter, it is common for all the conditions influencing an event such as premature birth to be interrelated. Thus, in the figure below, each cluster of arrows leading to an event reflects a network of factors that may have different causal relationships. Some possible examples are shown in Figure 4.

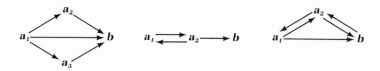

Figure 4 *Some possible patterns of multiple influences among points in a predictive chain.*

None of these figures is intended to be a complete or even accurate model of development, nor do we claim to have exhausted all the possibilities. Our purpose is primarily to illustrate the kind of complexity that seems to be necessary to account for developmental outcomes. One of the lessons we have learned from the attempt to isolate simple cause–effect relationships is that development is an extremely complex process. An adequate understanding of such a process requires models that are equally complex. This conclusion is not unique to the study of premature birth. Longitudinal research on children born at term has also been relatively unsuccessful in documenting simple cause–effect relationships between early experiences and later development. Thus, research in all areas of development is increasingly guided by more complex models of the developmental process.

The study of children born prematurely can continue to be illuminating in this endeavor. We noted in Chapter 2 that developmental outcomes following preterm birth seem to encompass the same range of variations that we see in the full-term population. Medical concern about the outcome of preterm birth has led to the collection of extensive data on all aspects of development for the preterm population, while comparable information for most of the full-term population is lacking. In this way, a data pool has been created that may be of use in answering general questions about development as well as specific questions concerned with preterm birth.

When we turn to the data on development of preterm infants, there is very little evidence that premature birth in and of itself has enduring effects on development. In Chapters 2 and 3, we found that, in some respects, early birth was associated with a small, but transient advantage in development. The curves for the data in Figure 2 in Chapter 3 (p. 56) were one example of this. Acceleration in development of a preference for three-dimensional over two-dimensional stimuli (Chapter 3) was another example. More often, early birth seemed to be associated with some disadvantages such as delayed motor development (Chapter 2), less efficient information processing (Chapter 3), and a more difficult temperament (Chapter 4).

However, one of the most consistent findings is that the rate of development was generally unaffected by premature birth (Chapters 2 and 4). That is, the rate of development seems to depend on underlying maturational processes that are progressing on a preset schedule that continues to unfold whether the infant is in the womb or in an incubator. However, because we are so accustomed to dating age from birth (rather than from conception, as discussed in Chapter 2), it usually appears that the preterm infant is lagging behind her age mates. Often this is because we have been using the wrong age mates. When we choose infants of the same age from term, the development of the preterm infant is more nearly on target, with much individual variation. Of course, if you are the parent, this knowledge may not make it any more pleasant to wait an extra two months for your baby's first smile or your first full night of sleep. But it does help to know that these apparent delays are normal for preterm infants.

The fact that preterm infants are, for the most part, indistinguishable from the general population after their early years suggests some other important features that are characteristics of the developmental process. First, it suggests that there is more than one path to the same outcome. Chapters 5 and 6 provided numerous examples of adults behaving differently toward preterm and full-term infants to produce the same result. For example, in feeding the very young preterm infant, who is easily overloaded by social stimulation, food intake may be maximized by engaging in as little social interaction as possible during feedings. For the full-term infant, a pleasant social exchange may make feedings more enjoyable and increase intake.

Another example is the study cited in Chapter 5, in which preterm and full-term infants did not differ in response to mothers' hiding games, but styles of mother–infant interaction did differ in the two groups. One explanation of this finding is that mother–infant interaction has nothing to do with the infant's understanding of permanence as an attribute of people. However, this seems unlikely. An alternative explanation is that each group of mothers adopted a style of interaction appropriate to infant development, with each group of infants having somewhat different needs. In Chapter 6, it was also suggested that some of the handicaps associated with preterm birth may be overcome or avoided by appropriate interventions.

An important and optimistic inference that can be made from much of the literature that we have reviewed is that development seems to have many built-in self-correcting features. At the beginning of this chapter, we listed some of the detrimental conditions associated with preterm birth and suggested that, in and of itself, such a list would lead one to a very pessimistic prognosis for development. While there are certainly some children for whom such pessimism is warranted, the more remarkable finding is that, despite so many threats to development, the majority of preterm infants do well. Several years after birth, they cannot be distinguished from their full-term age mates. To be sure, some of the credit goes to modern medical technology, which continues to make improvements in the early care of these children. Some of the credit must go to parents and families, who learn to cope with the additional stresses they face. Some of the credit must also go to practitioners in various support services who help parents to minimize or avoid potential problems. Finally, much of the credit must go to the apparent self-correcting nature of the developmental process and to the remarkable resiliency of the human infant.

Notes

Introduction

1. Henig, 1981.
2. Field et al., 1977.
3. For a more detailed history of preterm care, see Klaus and Kennell, 1976.
4. Budin, 1907.
5. Liebling, 1939.
6. Hess, Mohr, and Bartelme, 1934.
7. Hess and Lundeen, 1941.
8. Hess, Mohr, and Bartelme, 1934.
9. Osofsky and Kendall, 1977.
10. Selye, 1957.
11. Schwartz and Schwartz, 1977.
12. Drillien, 1964.
13. Kopp and Parmelee, 1979.

Chapter 1

1. Gordon, 1954; Patz, Hoeck, and dela Cruz, 1952.

2. Lubchenco et al., 1972. More recent studies suggest that, with the survival of younger and smaller babies who are vulnerable to retrolental fibroplasia for

other reasons, rates of retinal damage may again be increasing: Gunn et al., 1980.

3. Prince, Firlej, and Harvey, 1978.
4. Cornell and Gottfried, 1976.
5. Parmelee, 1979.
6. Some of the studies on which this view is based are Cravioto and Robles, 1965; Winick, 1968.
7. Lawson, Daum, and Turkewitz, 1977.
8. Speidel, 1978.
9. Terres, 1979.
10. Corter et al., 1978.
11. Minde et al., 1975.
12. Cornell and Gottfried, 1976.
13. Fanaroff, Kennell, and Klaus, 1972.
14. DiVitto and Goldberg, 1979.
15. Hawthorne, Richards, and Callon, 1978.
16. Herzog, 1979.
17. Parmelee, 1979.

Chapter 2

1. Bayley, 1969.
2. Appleton, Clifton, and Goldberg, 1975.
3. Bayley, 1965.
4. Cobb, Goodwin, and Saelens, 1966; Honzik, 1962; Klatskin, 1952; Klatskin, Jackson, and Wilkin, 1956.
5. Brazelton, 1973.
6. Rosenblith, 1961.
7. There are several places where you can find tables of developmental milestones: Caplan, 1978, 1980; Apgar and Beck, 1972, pp. 360–366; Cunningham and Sloper, 1980, Chap. 4. The latter two books may be of

special interest to parents whose preterm infant has a known or suspected handicap.

8. Brachfeld and Goldberg, 1978.
9. Hunt and Rhodes, 1977; Fitzhardinge et al., 1976.
10. L. Fetters, personal communication, 1980.
11. Drillien, 1964; Knobloch et al., 1956.
12. Kopp and Parmelee, 1979.
13. Field, Dempsey, and Shuman, 1979.
14. Caputo, Goldstein, and Taub, 1979.
15. Ehrlich et al., 1974.
16. Field, Dempsey, and Shuman, 1979.
17. Balow, Rubin, and Rosen, 1975–1976; Francis-Williams and Davies, 1974.
18. Drillien, 1972; Dweck et al., 1973.
19. Goldberg, 1981.
20. Goldberg, 1981.
21. Parmelee, Kopp, and Sigman, 1976.
22. Sigman and Parmelee, 1979.
23. Sameroff and Chandler, 1975.
24. Beckwith et al., 1976; Beckwith and Cohen, 1980; Cohen and Beckwith, 1979.

Chapter 3

1. McFarlane, 1975.
2. Fantz, 1956, 1958, 1965.
3. Parmelee, 1976.
4. Miranda and Hack, 1979.
5. Gesell and Amatruda, 1945; Saint–Anne Dargassies, 1966.
6. Hack, Mostow, and Miranda, 1976.
7. Miranda, 1970, 1976.
8. Kopp and Parmelee, 1979.

9. Parmelee, 1981; Parmelee and Sigman, 1976.
10. Sigman et al., 1977.
11. Lewis, Goldberg, and Campbell, 1969.
12. Sigman et al., 1977.
13. Fantz, Fagan, and Miranda, 1975.
14. Rose, 1980.
15. Schulman-Galambos and Galambos, 1979.
16. Hernandez, 1981.
17. Field et al., 1979; Rose, Schmidt, and Bridger, 1976.
18. Parmelee and Sigman, 1976.
19. Sigman, 1976.
20. Rose, Gottfried, and Bridger, 1978.
21. Fenson et al., 1976; McCall, 1974.
22. Jackowitz and Watson, 1980.
23. Kopp, 1976.
24. Brachfeld, Goldberg, and Sloman, 1980.
25. Graham, Matarazzo, and Caldwell, 1956; Rosenblith, 1966, 1975.
26. Miranda and Hack, 1979.
27. Kearsley, 1979.
28. Sameroff, 1981.
29. Sigman, Cohen, and Forsythe, 1981.

Chapter 4

1. Lorenz, 1943.
2. Korner and Grobstein, 1966.
3. Ter Vrught and Pederson, 1973.
4. Stern, 1974.
5. Freedman, 1974; Bowlby, 1969.
6. Freedman, 1974.
7. Foley, 1977.
8. Crow and Gowers, 1979.

9. Lester and Zeskind, 1979.
10. Frodi et al., 1978.
11. DiVitto and Goldberg, 1979; Field, 1979; Sostek, Quinn, and Davitt, 1979.
12. DiVitto and Goldberg, 1979.
13. Field, 1977.
14. Crawford, 1982.
15. Brachfeld, Goldberg, and Sloman, 1980.
16. Field, 1979.
17. Crawford, 1982.
18. Field, 1977; Brachfeld, Goldberg, and Sloman, 1980.
19. DiVitto and Goldberg, 1979; Field, 1977; Sostek, Quinn, and Davitt, 1979.
20. Field et al., 1978.
21. Field, 1979.
22. Brown and Bakeman, 1979.
23. DiVitto and Goldberg, in press.
24. Brachfeld, Goldberg, and Sloman, 1980.
25. Crawford, 1982.
26. Goldberg, Brachfeld, and DiVitto, 1980.
27. Ainsworth et al., 1978.
28. Field, Dempsey, and Shuman, 1979; Brown and Bakeman, 1980; Hock, Coady, and Cordero, 1973; Rode et al., 1981.
29. Field, Dempsey, and Shuman, 1979.
30. Brown and Bakeman, 1980.

Chapter 5

1. Herzog, 1980.
2. Personal communication, 1975.
3. Klaus and Kennell, 1976.
4. Caplan, 1960.

5. Personal communication, 1975.
6. DiVitto and Goldberg, 1979.
7. DiVitto and Goldberg, 1979.
8. DiVitto and Goldberg, 1979.
9. Kaplan and Mason, 1960.
10. Klaus and Kennell, 1976.
11. Seashore et al., 1973.
12. Klaus and Kennell, 1976, p. 14.
13. Klaus and Kennell, 1982.
14. Goldberg, 1982; Leiderman, 1982.
15. Barnett et al., 1970.
16. Kennell, Trause, and Klaus, 1975.
17. Leifer et al., 1972.
18. Kennell, Trause, and Klaus, 1975.
19. Auerbach, 1977.
20. Goldberg, 1979b; Klaus and Kennell, 1976.
21. Sameroff and Chandler, 1975.
22. Elmer and Gregg, 1967; Goldson et al., 1978; Klein and Stern, 1971; Shaheen et al., 1968.
23. Field, 1977.
24. Goldberg, 1978.
25. Leifer et al., 1972.
26. Fanaroff, Kennell, and Klaus, 1972.
27. DiVitto and Goldberg, 1979; Klaus et al., 1970; Leifer et al., 1972.
28. DiVitto and Goldberg, 1979.
29. Brachfeld, Goldberg, and Sloman, 1980.
30. Beckwith and Cohen, 1978.
31. Brown and Bakeman, 1979.
32. Schweitzer, 1979.
33. Field, 1977.
34. Personal communication, 1976.

35. Wasserman et al., 1980.
36. Goldberg, 1979a, 1982.
37. Sander, 1975.

Chapter 6

1. Neal, 1968.
2. Barnard, 1972.
3. Korner et al., 1975.
4. Kraemer and Pierpoint, 1976.
5. Hasselmeyer, 1964.
6. Freedman, Boverman, and Freedman, 1966; White and Labarba, 1976.
7. Solkoff et al., 1969.
8. White and Labarba, 1976.
9. Solkoff and Matuszak, 1975.
10. Scarr-Salapatek and Williams, 1973.
11. Powell, 1974.
12. Rosenfield, 1980.
13. Minde et al., 1980.
14. DiVitto and Goldberg, 1979.
15. Personal communication, 1979.
16. Scarr-Salapatek and Williams, 1973.
17. Rice, 1977.
18. Bromwich and Parmelee, 1979.
19. Gorski, 1979.

Glossary

Acute Referring to an illness that is severe and of brief duration.

Aetiology *See* Etiology.

Amniotic Referring to the fluid in the sac that contains the fetus during prenatal development.

Apnea The absence of breathing.

Arousal The level of physiological and behavioral activity, ranging from low (deep sleep) to high (agitated crying).

Aspiration The sucking of fluid into the air passages.

Attachment An emotional bond, particularly the young child's emotional bond to his or her parents.

Auditory Referring to the ears or the process of hearing.

Auditory evoked potentials Electrical signals recorded from auditory centers in the brain in response to sounds.

Bilirubin A substance produced by the breakdown of red blood cells.

Birth order Position in the family; for example, first born, last born.

Bonding The process of forming an emotional attachment; sometimes used to describe rapid and irreversible changes in parental feelings about a new infant, thought to occur in the first few hours of the infant's life.

Bradycardia A slowing of heartbeats.

Bronchopulmonary dysplasia (BPD) A condition in which there are abnormal changes in lung tissue.

Cardiac Referring to the heart.

Caretaking casualty A child suffering from inadequate or abusive care.

Chronic Referring to an illness of long duration.

Circulatory system The network, consisting of the heart and blood vessels, that allows blood to reach all organs of the body.

Cognitive Referring to thought processes or mental activity (cognition).

Discrepancy method A method of testing sensory, perceptual, or cognitive processes, in which a single stimulus is repeated and then followed by the presentation of a new stimulus or a variant of the original stimulus.

Dishabituation The increase in attention when a new stimulus or event is introduced after repetitions of an old stimulus or event. *See also* Habituation.

Dyad A pair.

Embryo The unborn infant from conception to the eighth week. *See also* Fetus.

Endogenous Referring to origin within the body.

Etiology The cause or origin (of disease).

Fetus   The unborn infant from the eighth week following conception to birth. *See also* Embryo.

Gavage   Feeding by a tube passed through the nose to the stomach.

Gestation   Pregnancy.

Habituation   The decrease in attention, associated with repetitions of an event or a stimulus. *See also* Dishabituation.

Hemorrhage   Bleeding (especially, heavy bleeding).

Humidity   Moisture or dampness (especially, of the air).

Hyperbilirubinemia   A condition in which too much bilirubin is present in the blood; jaundice.

Iatrogenic   Referring to a condition resulting from treatment.

Intravenous   Referring to, for example, feedings or injections introduced into a vein.

Intraventricular hemorrhage (IVH)   Bleeding into the brain.

Intubation   The insertion of a tube (for feeding, assistance in breathing, and the like).

Jaundice   *See* Hyperbilirubinemia.

Kinesthetic   Referring to the sense perception of movement.

Kwashiorkor   A severe form of malnutrition in which there is a shortage of protein as well as of the total amount of food.

Longitudinal   Referring to a study in which the same group of individuals is tested repeatedly as they get older.

Miscarriage   The spontaneous delivery before the sixth month of pregnancy.

Neonatology   The study of diseases of the newborn.

Neurological   Referring to the nervous system.

NICU (neonatal intensive-care unit)   A hospital unit specializing in the care of seriously ill newborns.

Object permanence   The concept that objects exist independently of our sensory contact with them; infants usually acquire this concept late in the first year. *See also* Person permanence.

Olfaction   The sense of smell.

Orienting response   A pattern of physical and behavioral changes characteristic of attention to novel or unexpected events (for example, interrupting ongoing activity, decrease in heart rate, turning toward a stimulus).

Parity   The number of births (live or stillborn) that a woman has experienced.

Patterned stimulation   Stimulation that is organized and regular in appearance, timing, frequency, and the like (for example, regular changes of light and dark accompanying day-night cycles).

Perceptual   Referring to the way incoming sensory information is interpreted by the brain (perception).

Perinatal   Occurring during or around the time of birth.

Person permanence   The concept that people exist independently of our sensory contact with them; most infants acquire this concept before object permanence. *See also* Object permanence.

Placenta The organ that directly connects the fetus with the mother during prenatal development; food and oxygen are delivered to the fetus, and waste products removed, by the placenta. *See also* Umbilical cord.

Postnatal age Age calculated from the time of birth.

Postterm age Age calculated from the expected date of birth.

Premature Referring to a birth that occurs before 37 weeks from conception; full-term gestation is 38–42 weeks from conception.

Prognosis The forecast of outcome.

Reflex An involuntary behavior involving a simple response to stimulation.

Respirator An apparatus that administers artificial respiration.

Respiratory distress syndrome (RDS) The inability to breathe adequately, caused by immaturity of the lungs in preterm infants.

Retina A layer of cells at the back part of the eyeball that is sensitive to light.

Retrolental fibroplasia The abnormal increase of fibrous tissue behind the lens of the eye.

Rooting A reflex behavior in which the newborn turns toward a touch on the cheek.

Sequelae Conditions that follow as a consequence of disease.

Small-for-dates Underweight for age at birth.

Spontaneous abortion The spontaneous delivery before the fetus is viable.

Standardization sample   The group on which norms for a test are developed.

Startle response   The response to sudden or loud noise or sudden loss of physical support.

Syndrome   A cluster of symptoms occurring together, recognizable as a disease.

Tactile   Referring to the sense of touch.

Transfusion   The transfer of blood from one person to another.

Trauma   Injury.

Umbilical cord   The structure projecting from the navel connecting the fetus to the placenta during pregnancy. *See also* Placenta.

Uterus   The muscular organ inside which the unborn infant develops during pregnancy.

Ventilator   An apparatus that assists breathing.

Wet nurse   A woman other than the mother who breast-feeds a baby.

Bibliography

Ainsworth, M. D. S., M. C. Blehar, E. Waters, and S. Wall. 1978. *Patterns of Attachment*. Hillsdale, N.J.: Lawrence Erlbaum Associates.

Anthony, E. (Ed.). 1975. *Explorations in Child Psychiatry*. New York: Plenum.

Apgar, V., and J. Beck. 1972. *Is My Baby All Right?* New York: Pocket Books.

Appleton, T., R. Clifton, and S. Goldberg. 1975. "The Development of Behavioral Competence in Infancy." In F. D. Horowitz (Ed.), *Review of Child Development Research*. Vol. 4. Chicago: University of Chicago Press.

Auerbach, K. 1977. "Breast Feeding the Premature Infant." *Keeping Abreast Journal, 11*, 98–119.

Balow, R., R. Rubin, and M. J. Rosen. 1975–1976. "Perinatal Events as Precursors of Reading Disability." *Reading Research Quarterly, 11*, 36–71.

Barnard, K. E. 1972. "The Effect of Stimulation on the Duration and Amount of Sleep and Wakefulness in the Premature Infant." Unpublished doctoral dissertation, University of Washington.

Barnett, C. R., P. H. Leiderman, R. Grobstein, and M. H. Klaus. 1970. "Neonatal Separation: The Maternal Side of Interactional Deprivation." *Pediatrics, 45,* 197–205.

Bayley, N. 1965. "Comparisons of Mental and Motor Tests for Ages 1–15 Months by Sex, Birth Order, Race, Geographical Location and Education of Parents." *Child Development, 36,* 379–411.

Bayley, N. 1969. *The Bayley Scales of Infant Development.* New York: Psychological Corporation.

Beckwith, L., and S. E. Cohen. 1978. "Preterm Birth: Hazardous Obstetrical and Postnatal Events as Related to Caregiver–Infant Behavior." *Infant Behavior and Development, 1,* 403–412.

Beckwith, L., and S. E. Cohen. 1980. "Interactions of Preterm Infants." In T. Field, S. Goldberg, D. Stern, and A. Sostek (Eds.), *High-Risk Infants and Children: Adult and Peer Interactions.* New York: Academic Press.

Beckwith, L., S. E. Cohen, C. B. Kopp, A. H. Parmelee, and T. G. March. 1976. "Caregiver–Infant Interaction and Early Cognitive Development in Preterm Infants." *Child Development, 47,* 579–587.

Bell, R. W., and W. P. Smotherman (Eds.). 1979. *Maternal Influences and Early Behavior.* Jamaica, N.Y.: Spectrum.

Bowlby, J. 1969. *Attachment and Loss.* Vol. 1: *Attachment.* New York: Basic Books.

Brachfeld, S., and S. Goldberg. 1978. "Parent–Infant Interaction: Effects of Newborn Medical Status on Free Play at 8 and 12 Months." Paper presented at the Southeastern Conference on Human Development, Atlanta.

Brachfeld, S., S. Goldberg, and J. Sloman. 1980. "Parent–Infant Interaction in Free Play at 8 and 12 months: Effects of Prematurity and Immaturity." *Infant Behavior and Development, 3,* 289–305.

Brazelton, T. B. 1973. *The Brazelton Neonatal Behavioral Assessment Scales.* Clinics in Developmental Medicine No. 50. Philadelphia: Lippincott.

Brimblecombe, F. S. W., M. P. M. Richards, and N. R. C. Roberton (Eds.). 1978. *Separation and Special Care Baby Units.* London: Spastics International Medical Publications/Heinemann.

Bromwich, R. M., and A. H. Parmelee. 1979. "An Intervention Program for Preterm Infants." In T. M. Field, A. M. Sostek, S. Goldberg, and H. H. Shuman (Eds.), *Infants Born at Risk.* Jamaica, N.Y.: Spectrum.

Brown, J. V., and R. Bakeman. 1979. "Relationships of Human Mothers with Their Infants During the First Year of Life." In R. W. Bell and W. P. Smotherman (Eds.), *Maternal Influences and Early Behavior.* Jamaica, N.Y.: Spectrum.

Brown, J. V., and R. Bakeman. 1980. "Early Interaction: Consequences for Social and Mental Development at 3 Years." *Child Development, 51,* 437–447.

Budin, P. 1907. *The Nursling.* London: Caxton.

Caplan, F. (Ed.). 1978. *The First Twelve Months of Life.* Des Plaines, Ill.: Bantam Books.

Caplan, F. (Ed.). 1980. *The Second Twelve Months of Life.* Des Plaines, Ill.: Bantam Books.

Caplan, G. 1960. "Patterns of Parental Response to the Crisis of Premature Birth." *Psychiatry, 23,* 365–374.

Caputo, D. V., K. M. Goldstein, and H. B. Taub. 1979. "The Development of Prematurely Born Children Through Middle Childhood." In T. M. Field, A. M. Sostek, S. Goldberg, and H. H. Shuman (Eds.), *Infants Born at Risk.* Jamaica, N.Y.: Spectrum.

Cobb, K., R. Goodwin, and E. Saelens. 1966. "Spontaneous Hand Positions of Newborn Infants." *Journal of Genetic Psychology, 108,* 225–237.

Cohen, L. B., and P. Salapatek (Eds.). 1975. *Infant Perception: From Sensation to Cognition.* Vol. 1. New York: Academic Press.

Cohen, S. E., and L. Beckwith. 1979. "Preterm Infant Interaction with the Caregiver in the First Year of Life and Competence at Age Two." *Child Development, 50,* 767–776.

Cornell, E. H., and A. W. Gottfried. 1976. "Intervention with Preterm Infants." *Child Development, 47,* 32–39.

Corter, C., S. Trehub, C. Boukydis, L. Ford, L. Celhoffer, and K. Minde. 1978. "Nurses' Judgments of the Attractiveness of Preterm Infants." *Infant Behavior and Development, 1,* 373–380.

Cravioto, J., and B. Robles. 1965. "Evolution of Adaptive and Motor Behavior During Rehabilitation from Kwashiorkor." *American Journal of Orthopsychiatry, 35,* 449–464.

Crawford, J. W. 1982. "Mother–Infant Interaction in Premature and Full Term Infants." *Child Development, 53,* 957–962.

Crow, B. M., and J. I. Gowers. 1979. "The Smiling Age of Preterm Babies." *Developmental Medicine and Child Neurology, 21,* 174–177.

Cunningham, C., and P. Sloper. 1980. *Helping Your Exceptional Baby.* New York: Random House.

DiVitto, B., and S. Goldberg. 1979. "The Development of Early Parent–Infant Interaction as a Function of Newborn Medical Status." In T. M. Field, A. M. Sostek, S. Goldberg, and H. H. Shuman (Eds.), *Infants Born at Risk.* Jamaica, N.Y.: Spectrum.

DiVitto, B., and S. Goldberg. In press. "Talking and Sucking: Infant Feeding Behavior and Parent Stimulation in Dyads with Different Medical Histories." *Infant Behavior and Development.*

Drillien, C. M. 1964. *The Growth and Development of the Prematurely Born Infant.* Edinburgh: Livingstone.

Drillien, C. M. 1972. "Aetiology and Outcome in Low Birthweight Infants." *Developmental Medicine and Child Neurology, 14,* 563–574.

Dweck, H. S., S. A. Saxon, J. W. Benton, and G. Casady. 1973. "Early Development of the Tiny Preterm Infant." *American Journal of Diseases of Childhood, 126,* 28–34.

Ehrlich, C., E. Shapiro, B. Kimball, and M. Huttner. 1974. "Communication Skills in 5-Year-Old Children with High Risk Newborn Histories." *Journal of Speech and Hearing Research, 16,* 522–529.

Elmer, E., and G. S. Gregg. 1967. "Developmental Characteristics of Abused Children." *Pediatrics, 40,* 596–602.

Falkner, F. (Ed.). 1966. *Human Development*. Philadelphia: Saunders.

Fanaroff, A. A., J. H. Kennell, and M. H. Klaus. 1972. "Follow-Up of Low Birthweight Infants—The Predictive Value of Maternal Visiting Patterns." *Pediatrics, 49*, 287–290.

Fantz, R. L. 1956. "A Method for Studying Early Visual Development." *Perceptual and Motor Skills, 6*, 13–15.

Fantz, R. L. 1958. "Pattern Vision in Young Infants." *Psychological Record, 8*, 43–47.

Fantz, R. L. 1965. "Visual Perception from Birth as Shown by Pattern Selectivity." In H. E. Whipple (Ed.), *New Issues in Infant Development. Annals of the New York Academy of Science, 118*, 793–814.

Fantz, R. L., J. F. Fagan, and S. B. Miranda. 1975. "Early Visual Selectivity." In L. B. Cohen and P. Salapatek (Eds.), *Infant Perception: From Sensation to Cognition.* Vol. 1. New York: Academic Press.

Fenson, L., J. Kagan, R. B. Kearsley, and P. R. Zelazo. 1976. "The Developmental Progression of Manipulative Play in the First Two Years." *Child Development, 47*, 232–236.

Field, T. 1977. "Effects of Early Separation, Interactive Deficits, and Experimental Manipulation on Mother–Infant Interaction." *Child Development, 48*, 763–771.

Field, T. 1979. "Interaction Patterns of Preterm and Full Term Infants." In T. M. Field, A. M. Sostek, S. Goldberg, and H. H. Shuman (Eds.), *Infants Born at Risk.* Jamaica, N.Y.: Spectrum.

Field, T., C. Dabiri, N. Hallock, and H. H. Shuman. 1977. "Developmental Effects of Prolonged Pregnancy and the Postmaturity Syndrome." *Journal of Pediatrics, 90,* 836–839.

Field, T. M., J. R. Dempsey, J. Hatch, G. Ting, and R. K. Clifton. 1979. "Cardiac and Behavioral Responses to Repeated Tactile and Auditory Stimulation by Preterm and Term Neonates." *Developmental Psychology, 15,* 406–416.

Field, T. M., J. R. Dempsey, and H. H. Shuman. 1979. "Developmental Assessments of Infants Surviving the Respiratory Distress Syndrome." In T. M. Field, A. M. Sostek, S. Goldberg, and H. H. Shuman (Eds.), *Infants Born at Risk.* Jamaica, N.Y.: Spectrum.

Field, T., S. Goldberg, D. Stern, and A. Sostek (Eds.). 1980. *High-Risk Infants and Children: Adult and Peer Interactions.* New York: Academic Press.

Field, T., N. Hallock, J. Dempsey, and H. H. Shuman. 1978. "Mothers' Assessments of Term and Pre-term Infants with RDS." *Child Psychiatry and Human Development, 9,* 75–85.

Field, T. M., A. M. Sostek, S. Goldberg, and H. H. Shuman (Eds.). 1979. *Infants Born at Risk.* Jamaica, N.Y.: Spectrum.

Fitzhardinge, P. M., K. Pape, M. Arstikaitis, M. Boyle, S. Ashby, A. Rowley, C. Netley, and P. R. Swyer. 1976. "Mechanical Ventilation of Infants of Less Than 1501 gm Birth Weight: Health, Growth, and Neurological Sequelae." *Journal of Pediatrics, 88,* 531–541.

Foley, H. 1977. "When Do Preterm and Small-for-Dates Babies Smile?" *Developmental Medicine and Child Neurology, 19,* 757–760.

Francis-Williams, J., and P. A. Davies. 1974. "Very Low Birthweight and Later Intelligence." *Developmental Medicine and Child Neurology, 16,* 709–728.

Freedman, D. G. 1974. *Human Infancy: An Evolutionary Perspective.* Hillsdale, N.J.: Lawrence Erlbaum Associates.

Freedman, D. G., H. Boverman, and N. Freedman. 1966. "Effects of Kinesthetic Stimulation on Weight Gain and Smiling in Premature Infants." Paper presented at the American Orthopsychiatric Association, San Francisco.

Friedlander, B. Z., G. M. Sterrit, and G. E. Kirk (Eds.). 1975. *Exceptional Infant.* Vol. 3: *Assessment and Intervention.* New York: Brunner/Mazel.

Friedman, S. L., and M. Sigman (Eds.). 1981. *Preterm Birth and Psychological Development.* New York: Academic Press.

Frodi, A., M. Lamb, L. Leavitt, C. Donovan, C. Neff, and D. Sherry. 1978. "Fathers' and Mothers' Response to the Faces and Cries of Normal and Premature Infants." *Developmental Psychology, 14,* 490–498.

Gesell, A., and C. S. Amatruda. 1945. *The Embryology of Behavior.* New York: Harper.

Goldberg, S. 1978. "Prematurity: Effects on Parent–Infant Interaction." *Journal of Pediatric Psychology, 3,* 137–144.

Goldberg, S. 1979a. "The Handicapped Infant and Compensatory Parenting." Paper presented at the

Keystone Conference on Parenting, Keystone, Colorado.

Goldberg, S. 1979b. "Pragmatics and Problems of Longitudinal Research with High Risk Infants." In T. M. Field, A. M. Sostek, S. Goldberg, and H. H. Shuman (Eds.), *Infants Born at Risk.* Jamaica, N.Y.: Spectrum.

Goldberg, S. 1981. *Cognitive and Motor Abilities of Preterm Infants.* Report to the National Foundation, March of Dimes.

Goldberg, S. 1982. "Some Biological Aspects of Early Parent–Infant Interaction." In S. G. Moore and C. R. Cooper (Eds.), *The Young Child: Reviews of Research.* Washington, D.C.: National Association for the Education of Young Children.

Goldberg, S., S. Brachfeld, and B. DiVitto. 1980. "Feeding, Fussing, and Play: Parent–Infant Interaction in the First Year as a Function of Prematurity and Perinatal Medical Problems." In T. Field, S. Goldberg, D. Stern, and A. Sostek (Eds.), *High-Risk Infants and Children: Adult and Peer Interactions.* New York: Academic Press.

Goldson, E., M. J. Fitch, T. H. Wendell, and G. Knapp. 1978. "Child Abuse: Its Relationship to Birthweight, Apgar Score and Developmental Testing." *American Journal of Diseases of Childhood, 132,* 790–793.

Gordon, H. H. 1954. "Oxygen Administration and Retrolental Fibroplasia." *Pediatrics, 14,* 543–546.

Gorski, P. 1979. Address presented at the Keystone Conference on Parenting, Keystone, Colorado.

Graham, F. D., R. G. Matarazzo, and B. M. Caldwell. 1956. "Behavioral Differences Between Normal and Traumatized Newborns." *Psychological Monographs, 70*(2), 427–438.

Gunn, T. R., J. Easdown, E. W. Outerbridge, and J. V. Aranda, 1980. "Risk Factors in Retrolental Fibroplasia." *Pediatrics, 65,* 1096–1100.

Hack, M., A. Mostow, and S. B. Miranda. 1976. "Development of Attention in Preterm Infants." *Pediatrics, 58,* 669–674.

Hasselmeyer, E. G. 1964. "The Premature Neonate's Response to Handling." *Journal of the American Nursing Association, 1,* 15–24.

Hawthorne, J. T., M. P. M. Richards, and M. Callon. 1978. "A Study of Parental Visiting of Babies in a Special-Care Unit." In F. S. W. Brimblecombe, M. P. M. Richards, and N. R. C. Roberton (Eds.), *Separation and Special Care Baby Units.* London: Spastics International Medical Publications/ Heinemann.

Henig, P. M. 1981. "The Child Savers." *New York Times,* March 22.

Hernandez, A. 1981. "Cardiac Orienting Response and Habituation/Dishabituation in Term and Preterm Infants to Pure Tone Auditory Stimuli." Paper presented at the Society for Research in Child Development, Boston.

Herzog, J. M. 1979. "Attachment, Attunement and Abuse: An Occurrence in Certain Preterm Infant–Parent Dyads and Triads." Paper presented at the American Academy of Child Psychiatry, Atlanta.

Herzog, J. 1980. A Neonatal Intensive Care Syndrome: A Pain Complex Involving Neuroplasticity and Psychic Trauma." Paper presented at the International Conference on Infant Psychiatry, Lisbon.

Hess, J. H., and E. C. Lundeen. 1941. *The Premature Infant.* Philadelphia: Lippincott.

Hess, J. H., G. J. Mohr, and P. F. Bartelme. 1934. *The Physical and Mental Growth of Prematurely Born Children.* Chicago: University of Chicago Press.

Hock, E., S. Coady, and L. Cordero. 1973. "Patterns of Attachment to Mother of One-Year-Old Infants." Paper presented at the Society for Research in Child Development, Philadelphia.

Honzik, M. 1962. *The Mental and Motor Test Performance for Suspected Brain Injury.* Final report contract SA43PH2426. Washington, D.C.: National Institutes of Health, National Institute of Neurological Diseases and Blindness, Collaborative Research.

Horowitz, F. D., E. M. Hetherington, S. Scarr-Salapatek, and G. Siegel (Eds.). 1975. *Review of Child Development Research.* Vol. 4. Chicago: University of Chicago Press.

Hunt, J. V., and L. Rhodes. 1977. "Mental Development of Preterm Infants During the First Year." *Child Development, 48,* 204–210.

Immelman, K., G. Barlow, M. Main, and L. Petrinovich (Eds.). 1982. *Issues in Behavioral Development: The Bielefeld Interdisciplinary Conference.* Cambridge, England: Cambridge University Press.

Jackowitz, E. R., and M. W. Watson. 1980. "Development of Object Transformations in Pretend Play." *Developmental Psychology, 16,* 543–549.

Kaplan, D. N., and E. H. Mason. 1960. "Maternal Reactions to Premature Birth Viewed as an Acute Emotional Disorder." *American Journal of Orthopsychiatry, 30,* 539–552.

Kearsley, R. 1979. "Iatrogenic Retardation: A Syndrome of Learned Incompetence." In R. B. Kearsley and I. E. Siegel (Eds.), *Infants at Risk: Assessment of Cognitive Functioning.* Hillsdale, N.J.: Lawrence Erlbaum Associates.

Kearsley, R. B., and I. E. Siegel (Eds.). 1979. *Infants at Risk: Assessment of Cognitive Functioning.* Hillsdale, N.J.: Lawrence Erlbaum Associates.

Kennell, J. H., M. A. Trause, and M. H. Klaus. 1975. "Evidence for a Sensitive Period in the Human Mother." In *Parent–Infant Interaction.* CIBA Foundation Symposium No. 33. Amsterdam: Elsevier.

Klatskin, E. H. 1952. "Intelligence Test Performance at One Year Among Infants Raised with Flexible Methodology." *Journal of Clinical Psychology, 8,* 230–237.

Klatskin, E. H., E. B. Jackson, and L. C. Wilkin. 1956. "The Influence of Degree of Flexibility in Maternal Child Care Practices on Early Child Behavior." *American Journal of Orthopsychiatry, 26,* 79–93.

Klaus, M. H., and J. H. Kennell. 1976. *Maternal–Infant Bonding.* St. Louis: Mosby.

Klaus, M. H., and J. H. Kennell. 1982. *Parent–Infant Bonding.* St. Louis: Mosby.

Klaus, M. H., J. H. Kennell, N. Plumb, and S. Zuelke. 1970. "Human Maternal Behavior at First Contact With Her Young." *Pediatrics, 46,* 187–192.

Klein, M., and L. Stern. 1971. "Low Birth Weight and the Battered Child Syndrome." *American Journal of Diseases of Childhood, 122,* 15–18.

Knobloch, H., R. Rider, P. Harper, and B. Pasamanick. 1956. "Neuropsychiatric Sequelae of Prematurity: A Longitudinal Study." *Journal of the American Medical Association, 161,* 581–585.

Kopp, C. 1976. "Action Schemas of 8-Month-Olds." *Developmental Psychology, 12,* 361–362.

Kopp, C. B., and A. H. Parmelee. 1979. "Prenatal and Perinatal Influences on Infant Behavior." In J. D. Osofsky (Eds.), *Handbook of Infant Development.* New York: Wiley.

Korner, A., and R. Grobstein. 1966. "Visual Alertness as Related to Soothing in Neonates: Implications for Material Stimulation and Early Deprivation." *Child Development, 37,* 867–876.

Korner, A. F., H. C. Kraemer, M. E. Faffner, and L. M. Cosper. 1975. "Effects of Waterbed Flotation on Premature Infants: A Pilot Study." *Pediatrics, 56,* 361–367.

Kraemer, H. C., and M. E. Pierpoint. 1976. "Rocking Waterbeds and Auditory Stimuli to Enhance Growth of Preterm Infants." *Journal of Pediatrics, 88,* 297–299.

Lawson, D., C. Daum, and G. Turkewitz. 1977. "Environmental Characteristics of a Neonatal Intensive Care Unit." *Child Development, 48,* 1633–1639.

Leiderman, P. H. 1982. "The Critical Period Hypothesis Revisited: Mother to Infant Social Bonding in the Neonatal Period." In K. Immelman, G. Barlow, M. Main, and L. Petrinovich (Eds.), *Issues in Behavioral Development: The Bielefeld Interdisciplinary Conference.* Cambridge, England: Cambridge University Press.

Leifer, A. D., P. H. Leiderman, C. R. Barnett, and J. A. Williams. 1972. "Effects of Mother–Infant Separation on Maternal Attachment Behavior." *Child Development, 43,* 1303–1318.

Lester, B. M., and P. S. Zeskind. 1979. "The Organization and Assessment of Crying in the Infant at Risk." In T. M. Field, A. M. Sostek, S. Goldberg, and H. H. Shuman (Eds.), *Infants Born at Risk.* Jamaica, N.Y.: Spectrum.

Lewis, M., S. Goldberg, and H. Campbell. 1969. "A Developmental Study of Information Processing Within the First Three Years of Life." *Monographs of the Society for Research in Child Development, 34,* Serial No. 133.

Lewis, M., and L. A. Rosenblum (Eds.). 1974. *The Effect of the Infant on Its Caregiver.* New York: Wiley.

Liebling, A. 1939. "Profiles: Patron of the Premies." *The New Yorker,* June 3, pp. 20–24.

Lorenz, K. 1943. "Die angeborenen Formen naglicher Erfahrung." *Zeitschrift Tierpsychologie, 5,* 235–409. Cited in E. Hess. "Ethology and Developmental Psychology." In P. H. Mussen (Ed.), *Carmichael's Manual of Child Psychology.* 3rd ed. New York: Wiley, 1970.

Lubchenco, L. O., M. Delivoria-Papadopoulos, L. J. Butterfield, J. H. French, D. Metcalf, I. E. Hix, J. Danick, J. Dodds, M. Downs, and E. Freeland. 1972. "Long-Term Followup Studies of Prematurely Born Infants. I: Relationship of Handicaps to Nursery Routines." *Journal of Pediatrics, 80,* 501–508.

McCall, R. B. 1974. "Exploratory Manipulation and Play in the Human Infant." *Monographs of the Society for Research in Child Development, 39,* Serial No. 155.

McFarlane, J. A. 1975. "Olfaction in the Development of Social Preferences in the Human Neonate. In *Parent–Infant Interaction.* CIBA Foundation Symposium No. 33. Amsterdam: Elsevier.

Minde, K., L. Ford, L. Celhoffer, and C. Boukydis. 1975. "Interactions of Mothers and Nurses with Preterm Infants." *Canadian Medical Association Journal, 113,* 741–745.

Minde, K., N. Shosenberg, P. Marton, J. Thompson, J. Ripley, and S. Burns. 1980. "Self-Help Groups in a Premature Nursery—A Controlled Evaluation." *Pediatrics, 96,* 933–940.

Miranda, S. B. 1970. "Visual Abilities and Pattern Preferences of Premature Infants and Full Term Neonates." *Journal of Experimental Child Psychology, 10,* 189–205.

Miranda, S. B. 1976. "Visual Attention in Defective and High Risk Infants." *Merrill–Palmer Quarterly, 22,* 201–228.

Miranda, S. B., and M. Hack. 1979. "The Predictive Value of Neonatal Visual–Perceptual Behaviors." In T. M.

Field, A. M. Sostek, S. Goldberg, and H. H. Shuman (Eds.), *Infants Born at Risk.* Jamaica, N.Y.: Spectrum.

Moore, S. G., and C. R. Cooper (Eds.). 1982. *The Young Child: Reviews of Research.* Washington, D.C.: National Association for the Education of Young Children.

Mussen, P. H. (Ed.). 1970. *Carmichael's Manual of Child Psychology.* 3rd ed. New York: Wiley.

Neal, M. 1968. "Vestibular Stimulation and Developmental Behavior of the Small Premature Infant." *Nursing Research Reports, 3,* 2–5.

Osofsky, J. D. (Ed.). 1979. *Handbook of Infant Development.* New York: Wiley.

Osofsky, H., and N. Kendall. 1977. "Poverty as a Criterion of Risk." In J. L. Schwartz and L. H. Schwartz (Eds.), *Vulnerable Infants,* New York: McGraw-Hill.

Parmelee, A. H. 1976. "Neurological and Behavioral Organization of Premature Infants in the First Months of Life." *Biological Psychiatry, 10,* 501–512.

Parmelee, A. H. 1979. "Discussion." In E. B. Thoman (Eds.), *Origins of the Infant's Social Responsiveness.* Hillsdale, N.J.: Lawrence Erlbaum Associates.

Parmelee, A. H. 1981. "Auditory Function and Neurological Maturation in Preterm Infants." In S. L. Friedman and M. Sigman (Eds.), *Preterm Birth and Psychological Development.* New York: Academic Press.

Parmelee, A. H., C. B. Kopp, and M. Sigman. 1976. "Selection of Developmental Assessment Techniques for Infants at Risk." *Merrill–Palmer Quarterly, 22,* 177–199.

Parmelee, A. H., and M. Sigman. 1976. "Development of Visual Behavior and Neurological Organization in Preterm and Full Term Infants." In A. D. Pick (Ed.), *Minnesota Symposium on Child Psychology*. Vol. 10. Minneapolis: University of Minnesota Press.

Patz, A. L., E. Hoeck, and E. dela Cruz. 1952. "Studies on the Effects of High Oxygen in Retrolental Fibroplasia. I: Nursery Observations." *American Journal of Ophthalmology, 35,* 1248–1252.

Pick, A. D. (Ed.). 1976. *Minnesota Symposium on Child Psychology*. Vol. 10. Minneapolis: University of Minnesota Press.

Powell, L. F. 1974. "The Effect of Extra Stimulation and Maternal Involvement on the Development of Low Birth Weight Infants and on Maternal Behavior." *Child Development, 45,* 106–113.

Prince, J., M. Firlej, and D. Harvey. 1978. "Contact Between Babies in Incubators and Their Caretakers." In F. S. W. Brimblecombe, M. P. M. Richards, and N. R. C. Roberton (Eds.), *Separation and Special Care Baby Units*. London: Spastics International Medical Publications/Heinemann.

Rice, R. 1977. "Neurophysiological Development in Premature Infants Following Stimulation." *Developmental Psychology, 13,* 69–76.

Rode, S. S., P. Chang, R. O. Fisch, and L. A. Sroufe. 1981. "Attachment Patterns of Infants Separated at Birth." *Developmental Psychology, 17,* 188–192.

Rose, S. A. 1980. "Enhancing Visual Recognition Memory in Preterm Infants." *Developmental Psychology, 16,* 85–92.

Rose, S. A., A. W. Gottfried, and W. H. Bridger. 1978. "Cross-Modal Transference in Infancy: Relationship with Prematurity and Socioeconomic Background." *Developmental Psychology, 14,* 643–652.

Rose, S. A., K. Schmidt, and W. H. Bridger. 1976. "Cardiac and Behavioral Responsivity to Tactile Stimulation in Premature and Full Term Infants." *Developmental Psychology, 12,* 311–320.

Rosenblith, J. F. 1961. "The Modified Graham Behavior Test for Neonates: Test–Retest Reliability, Normative Data, and Hypotheses for Future Work." *Biologia Neonatorum, 3,* 174–192.

Rosenblith, J. 1966. "Prognostic Value of Behavioral Assessment of Neonates." *Child Development, 37,* 623–631.

Rosenblith, J. 1975. "Prognostic Value of Neonatal Behavioral Tests." In B. Z. Friedlander, G. M. Sterrit, and G. E. Kirk (Eds.), *Exceptional Infant.* Vol. 3: *Assessment and Intervention.* New York: Brunner/Mazel.

Rosenfield, A. G. 1980. "Visiting in the Intensive Care Nursery." *Child Development, 51,* 939–941.

Saint-Anne Dargassies, S. 1966. "Neurological Maturation of the Premature Infant of 28 to 41 Weeks Gestational Age." In F. Falkner (Ed.), *Human Development.* Philadelphia: Saunders.

Sameroff, A. J. 1981. "Longitudinal Studies of Preterm Infants: A Review of Chapters 17–20." In S. L. Friedman and M. Sigman (Eds.), *Preterm Birth and Psychological Development.* New York: Academic Press.

Sameroff, A. J., and M. J. Chandler. 1975. "Reproductive Risk and the Continuum of Caretaking Casualty." In F. D. Horowitz, E. M. Hetherington, S. Scarr-Salapatek, and G. Siegel (Eds.), *Review of Child Development Research.* Vol. 4. Chicago: University of Chicago Press.

Sander, L. 1975. "Infant and Caretaking Environment: Investigation and Conceptualization of Adaptive Behavior in a System of Increasing Complexity." In E. Anthony (Ed.), *Explorations in Child Psychiatry.* New York: Plenum.

Scarr-Salapatek, S., and M. L. Williams. 1973. "The Effects of Early Stimulation on Low Birthweight Infants." *Child Development,* 44, 94–101.

Schulman-Galambos, C., and R. Galambos. 1979. "Assessment of Hearing." In T. M. Field, A. M. Sostek, S. Goldberg, and H. H. Shuman (Eds.), *Infants Born at Risk.* Jamaica, N.Y.: Spectrum.

Schwartz, J. L., and L. H. Schwartz (Eds.). 1977. *Vulnerable Infants.* New York: McGraw-Hill.

Schweitzer, T. 1979. "Object Permanence, Person Permanence and Mother–Infant Interaction in Full Term and Preterm 11-Month-Olds." Unpublished doctoral dissertation, Brandeis University.

Seashore, M. L., A. D. Leifer, C. E. Barnett, and P. H. Leiderman. 1973. "The Effects of Denial of Early Mother–Infant Interaction on Maternal Self-Confidence." *Journal of Personality and Social Psychology,* 26, 269–378.

Selye, H. 1957. *The Stress of Life.* New York: McGraw-Hill.

Shaheen, E., D. Alexander, M. Truskovsky, and G. Barbero. 1968. "Failure to Thrive: A Retrospective Profile." *Clinical Pediatrics, 7,* 255–261.

Sigman, M. 1976. "Early Development of Preterm and Full Term Infants: Exploratory Behavior in 8-Month-Olds." *Child Development, 47,* 606–612.

Sigman, M., S. E. Cohen, and A. B. Forsythe. 1981. "The Relation of Early Infant Measures to Later Development." In S. L. Friedman and M. Sigman (Eds.), *Preterm Birth and Psychological Development.* New York: Academic Press.

Sigman, M., C. B. Kopp, B. Littman, and A. H. Parmelee. 1977. "Infant Visual Attention in Relation to Birth Condition." *Developmental Psychology, 13,* 431–437.

Sigman, M., and A. H. Parmelee. 1979. "Longitudinal Evaluation of the Preterm Infant." In T. M. Field, A. M. Sostek, S. Goldberg, and H. H. Shuman (Eds.), *Infants Born at Risk.* Jamaica, N.Y.: Spectrum.

Solkoff, N., and D. Matuszak. 1975. "Tactile Stimulation and Behavioral Development Among Low Birthweight Infants." *Child Psychiatry and Human Development, 6,* 33–37.

Solkoff, N., S. Yaffe, D. Weintraub, and B. Blase. 1969. "Effects of Handling on the Subsequent Development of Premature Infants." *Developmental Psychology, 1,* 765–768.

Sostek, A., P. Quinn, and M. Davitt. 1979. "Behavioral Development and Neurologic Status of Premature and Full Term Infants with Varying Medical Complications." In T. M. Field, A. M. Sostek, S. Goldberg, and H. H. Shuman (Eds.), *Infants Born at Risk.* Jamaica, N.Y.: Spectrum.

Speidel, B. D. 1978. "Adverse Effects of Routine Procedures on Preterm Infants." *Lancet,* April 22, pp. 564–566.

Stern, D. 1974. "Mother and Infant at Play: The Dyadic Interaction Involving Facial, Vocal and Gaze Behaviors." In M. Lewis and L. A. Rosenblum (Eds.), *The Effect of the Infant on Its Caregiver.* New York: Wiley.

Terres, N. 1979. "Psychological Aspects of Neonatal Intensive Care." Paper presented at the Fourth Annual Symposium on Clinical Applications of Research in Infant-Parent Relationships, Boston.

Ter Vrught, D., and D. Pederson. 1973. "The Effects of Vertical Rocking on the Arousal Level of Two-Month-Old Infants." *Child Development, 44,* 205–209.

Thoman, E. B. (Ed.). 1979. *Origins of the Infant's Social Responsiveness.* Hillsdale, N.J.: Lawrence Erlbaum Associates.

Wasserman, G., C. R. Solomon-Schwerzer, S. Spieker, and D. Stern. 1980. "Maternal Interactive Style with Normal and At-Risk Toddlers." Paper presented at the International Conference on Infant Studies, New Haven.

Whipple, H. E. (Ed.). 1965. *New Issues in Infant Development. Annals of the New York Academy of Sciences, 118.*

Index

DE